"Tender and tr

MW00565942

In *A Harvest From Pain*, Jane Grayshon presents an honest description of walking through unexplainable, unending and, most certainly, undeserved pain. She gives us permission to ask why, yet helps us learn to be content when no answer comes. Her writing is timely, tender and transparent.

Marilyn Heavilin
Author, *Roses in December* and
When Your Dreams Die

When the icy fingers of pain wrap themselves around us, we frequently look for a "spiritual band-aid" or a "way of escape." Neither of these were on God's agenda for Jane Grayshon. A "harvest" had to be produced. Like any harvest, something had to be cut down. Jane was. *A Harvest From Pain* will arrest your spirit and allow you to see the grace of God's sovereignty in a human life. I heartily recommend it for anyone.

Dr. James M. Christensen
President/Speaker
Heaven & Home Hour, Inc.

What a rich harvest gleaned from the life of Jane Grayshon! By sharing the depth of her personal suffering, she sows seeds of hope within us—hope that even the heaviest heart can be lifted to new heights by the loving hand of God.

June Hunt
Executive Director
Hope for the Heart

Also by Jane Grayshon

*A Pathway Through Pain: Pressing On
Despite Chronic Pain and Suffering*

Discovering God's Goodness
In the Midst of Your Suffering

A HARVEST FROM

Pain

JANE GRAYSHON

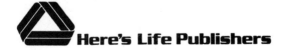
Here's Life Publishers

First Printing, September 1991

Published by
HERE'S LIFE PUBLISHERS, INC.
P. O. Box 1576
San Bernardino, CA 92402

© 1989, Jane Grayshon
North American edition published by special arrangement with
    Kingsway Publications, Eastbourne, England.
All rights reserved
Printed in the United States of America

Cover design by Cornerstone Graphics
Cover photography by Dennis Frates/Oregon Scenics

Library of Congress Cataloging-in-Publication Data
Grayshon, Jane.
    A harvest from pain : discovering God's goodness in the midst of your
suffering / Jane Grayshon.
        p.   cm.
    ISBN 0-89840-323-5
    1. Consolation. 2. Pain—Religious aspects—Christianity. 3. Suffering—
Religious aspects—Christianity. I. Title.
BV4905.2.G715   1991
248.8'6—dc20   91-627
                                                    CIP

    Unless indicated otherwise, Scripture quotations are from *The Holy Bible: New
International Version*, © 1973, 1978, 1984 by the International Bible Society.
Published by Zondervan Bible Publishers, Grand Rapids, Michigan. Scripture quota-
tions designated GNB are from *The Good News Bible*, © 1976, The American Bible
Society.

For More Information, Write:
L.I.F.E.—P.O. Box A399, Sydney South 2000, Australia
Campus Crusade for Christ of Canada—Box 300, Vancouver, B.C., V6C 2X3, Canada
Campus Crusade for Christ—Pearl Assurance House, 4 Temple Row, Birmingham, B2 5HG, England
Lay Institute for Evangelism—P.O. Box 8786, Auckland 3, New Zealand
Campus Crusade for Christ—P.O. Box 240, Raffles City Post Office, Singapore 9117
Great Commission Movement of Nigeria—P.O. Box 500, Jos, Plateau State Nigeria, West Africa
Campus Crusade for Christ International—Arrowhead Springs, San Bernardino, CA 92414, U.S.A.

To the Jocelyn
in all of us

Contents

As long as the earth endures,
seedtime and harvest . . .
will never cease
(Genesis 8:22).

Introduction

Three-quarters of the way through the writing of this book, a little blue memo appeared on my desk. Matthew's handwritten message was brief, almost cryptic: "The ancient harvest from pain!" (Psalm 119:71, NIV)

Thank you, Matthew, for that note, for sharing so generously and excitedly in the harvest as well as in the pain that has been ours together.

But I shudder with shame whenever I read the words of that verse. It reminds me of how very far short I fall in relating to my Father God. For only on rare days have I honestly been able to say with the psalmist, "It was good for me to be afflicted, so that I might learn your decrees."

Perhaps an evening like this, at the end of writing a book, might be one of those rare days. After an hour or so of quietness, of thinking and, occasionally, praying, I can bow myself before God and thank Him for teaching me His ways.

But when God doesn't *do* something to help us, it's all too easy to assume that He's more interested in bringing some virtue out of suffering than in caring about the suffering through which we learn! Forgive me, Lord, for mistaking Your nature. Many times I have insulted You in this way. May I always remember Your promise that Your goodness and steadfast love never cease—no matter how undeserved.

When pain slashes its way into my life, it causes me, and Matthew too, to feel cut through and ground down. It's hard to imagine that has anything to do with a harvest. Everything seems only a waste.

But harvesting is all about cutting and grinding down. And I cannot write of the awful, threshing pain without also saying that to escape that pain—something I often wish for—would be to escape God becoming bigger in me. And for that, I can truly thank Him.

I must also thank the hundreds of readers who, in writing to me in response to *A Pathway Through Pain,* have encouraged me to glimpse that there is always a harvest from pain, even if it is only for others to see. Many shared generously of their quiet pain: frail bodies, fragile minds, failing relationships, all hurt. There are so many silent sufferers. God knows. At times I have read of pain so grim, so black, it would have been glib to suggest that it might yield any harvest.

But with God, there is no death without resurrection. There is no suffering without the Father raising up. As at Easter, there is no stone covering even the darkest grave which He does not roll away, transforming it into a place of new beginnings, of fresh meeting with the Master, of renewed openness to His Spirit.

My prayer for you as you read this book is that you will glimpse God's Son as your close companion on your pathway through whatever pain you know — a companionship which is the most valuable harvest for which we can ever pray.

JANE GRAYSHON

All the people and places in this book are real, but some of the names and chronology of events have been changed in order to preserve anonymity. (Even my crossword-solving husband is still unraveling bits!)

1

Barriers Broken

People have put up a wall of loose stones
(Ezekiel 13:10, GNB).

"Jane!" The voice hailing me echoed around the street lined by Georgian houses.

I turned to search for the caller. As I did so, I caught the warmly familiar view which used to greet me every day on my way home from nursing in one of Edinburgh's big hospitals. The tall spires of the cathedral etched themselves against the horizon, reaching up to the clear sky above. It was good to see them again after having moved away to England. The years we had lived in Edinburgh had been especially happy.

"Jane!" I heard again, and the voice pulled me from my nostalgic reverie. I began to scan the street until behind a row of parked cars I caught sight of a figure waving to me. Almost instantly I recognized the smart suede jacket with its embroidered sleeves. It was Jocelyn.

She stepped sedately off the curb, turning her head only slightly to check the traffic. I smiled inwardly. She always maintained such poise; she seemed completely ordered and controlled.

Her step was deft and quick as she approached me. Not even the awkward cobblestones which composed the street in this part of the New Town caused her to lose her dignified manner. She held herself erect, unashamed of her tall figure which seemed so befitting to her high professional standing.

Her graying hair had been swept into a sleek bun which sat neatly at the nape of her neck. A few strands, blown by Edinburgh's east winds, had worked loose and now framed her face, softening it a little. Behind them, though, she still appeared the hospital matron I had always known her to be.

For a second I recoiled a little from her, foolishly daunted by her formidable appearance which I perceived as cold.

"Oh, good morning!" I smiled, surprised to meet her during so brief a visit back to our home city. I chose an appropriately polite greeting. Jocelyn was never casual.

I stopped and waited for her to catch up with me. I never had been completely at ease conversing with her. "How nice to see you," I added, rather nervously. She was such a gracious person herself, she elicited from me my most charming responses.

"How nice to see *you*," she replied. I watched her thin lips move as she spoke. *Does she ever accidentally smudge her lipstick,* I wondered irreverently, *or does she even get that perfect every time?*

We stood facing one another now. I was unsure of how to make conversation.

"How are you?" I asked automatically.

Jocelyn raised her hands as if to push away such irrelevant chitchat. It was a gesture signaling that she had not come over to discuss such niceties. "Oh, I'm fine," she replied. "Just fine."

Her hand, having returned immediately to rest back on the handle of her wicker shopping basket, fiddled a little impatiently. The basket squeaked in response.

"How are *you*?" she asked sincerely, frowning as if her own enquiry was much more relevant than mine. Her mouth softened into a smile whose sudden flicker of warmth surprised me.

"Oh," I laughed awkwardly. I did not know how to respond when people asked that of me. I found it an uncomfortable question. I could have replied in a number of ways. I could have told her of fairly major issues in my life, but I was not sure I was prepared to do that. It did not seem fitting with Jocelyn.

"I'm not bad," I replied evasively. I, too, did not intend to be dragged into a conversation which seemed irrelevant to our superficial meeting.

Her forehead puckered in puzzlement. Clearly she was frustrated to be tied to our usual formal politeness. She wanted to talk in more depth.

Jocelyn's gaze remained on me, her steely blue eyes unmoving. She was waiting for me to warm to her, but I was unsure how to do so.

Seeing my hesitation, Jocelyn spoke again.

"Your book . . . " she began.

Her tone suddenly alerted me.

"I've read it." She searched my face for me to lower my barriers of reticence.

I shuffled uneasily from one foot to the other and looked away. Was I expected to share more of myself than those who questioned me?

Jocelyn's frown settled on her forehead and she sighed. It was as if she was resigning herself to the fact that we were both too reticent to disclose matters which were close to our hearts.

It was then that she broke the ice. Her voice sounded almost begging, "Jane—why did you never tell me?"

It was my turn to frown now. Had she been hurt that she had not been the one in whom I had confided about my illness? Disappointed in me for not having trusted her? Angry at me for excluding her?

"It was a revelation to me," she tried to explain. "I had no idea your pain had been like that. I just never knew . . . " Her voice trailed away pensively.

Part of me wanted to reassure her, "Oh well, it wasn't too bad, and it's all over now." But that would not have been true. My illness had been every bit as bad as I had described. And after eleven years, there was nothing to suggest that the pain, the inflammation, the recurrent infections, the operations, would suddenly all be over.

In any case, I could see that Jocelyn would not have accepted such evasive assurances. Her uncompromising directness, though catching me off-guard, also invoked my confidence.

"But, Jocelyn, wait a minute," I began. "You did know a bit . . . "

"Not the *extent* of your pain," she countered while I was still speaking. "I had no idea of that."

Embarrassed, I avoided her gaze.

"I mean, I knew you had bad spells, and of course I knew whenever you were in the hospital but . . . " Her face contorted, as if she shared for a moment in the agony which she had read about.

My discomfort increased. "Well, I'm sorry," I apologized. "I find it very difficult. It's part of how I'm made. I just can't go around bemoaning how I feel. I'm terrified of being a boring, moaning woman. Perhaps it's all pride, lest I be seen as weak, or fear of other's reactions . . . " I checked myself, remembering who I was talking to. "Anyway, what difference would it have made?"

Jocelyn drew back a little and pushed the wandering strand of hair away from her eyes.

"What difference?" she repeated, astonished that I should ask so naive a question. "Why, I should have done so much more!"

I shook my head and smiled. "No," I said slowly. "No, Jocelyn, you shouldn't. What more could you have done?" I began to fidget. Perhaps, after all, this conversation was less profound than had at first seemed.

"Well," Jocelyn hesitated awkwardly, "I'm sure there's an awful lot I could have done." She gazed distantly down the street, as if seeking inspiration. "I could have—well, just come to see how you were

. . . made you cups of tea . . . brought you some home-baked goods."

"Yes," I began to warm to her suggestions. I had never imagined her to take time to show such tender gestures.

Immediately I felt guilty. I had prejudged her, apparently quite wrongly. I had taken her as she seemed rather than looking behind her appearance.

She was looking at me now, waiting for me to be more contrite, I imagined.

"I suppose I never thought you would have done that for me," I dared to say. I looked up at her, relieved to have been brave enough to be honest. Somehow it felt appropriate. I felt much closer to her even in such an unexpected conversation. Yet I was also slightly anxious because such affinity with her was so new and, ironically, almost alien.

I had no need to fear. Jocelyn's face melted into a warmly understanding smile, indicating an awareness of herself which astonished me. She knew how other people perceived her. Her eyes closed gently as she assented.

"Mmmm," she agreed. "And I don't suppose I gave you enough clues so that you could know." She hugged her creaky basket more closely to her.

So she did know herself! Underneath that side of her which I had assumed to be unfeeling and cold, she cared more deeply than I had ever guessed. Guilt swept over me as I thought how I had misunderstood her.

"Anyway," my fidgeting increased, "I'm terribly sorry, but I'm meeting Matthew in a minute, and I don't want to keep him waiting. It's a pity, though."

It was the first time I had ever felt like this. "I wish we could talk a bit more."

Jocelyn turned to walk back across the road, but hesitated. "There's more to say," she said, and I flinched a little at her formal-sounding voice once again. It seemed that there had been only the tiniest chink in her armor, and she had just closed it over.

What was the "more" she was thinking of? I wondered. I sensed that there was something on her mind. Something, perhaps, that she had not disclosed before.

As the wind whipped our faces, she turned to face me again. "Saturday?" she spoke questioningly. "I don't suppose you're going, are you?"

I thought for a second. Saturday? "Ah, the party?" Neither of us wanted to be first to name the special anniversary celebration, lest the other had not been invited.

Jocelyn nodded knowingly, then her eyes twinkled as she realized we would both be going. "I'll see you there," she tossed over her shoulder as she stepped out onto the cobblestones again.

"All right, then," I called after her. I sighed, amused. She was a different sort of lady from most of my friends. Of course, I had always admired her. But I was beginning to see her differently. I could warm to her in a way I would never have imagined possible.

Matthew was waiting for me by the floral clock of Princes Street Gardens. As I caught sight of the road behind him, distinctively coiling its way up The Mound from Princes Street, a thrill came over me.

During my first years as a student nurse, I had raced down that hill every Monday evening after my orchestral rehearsals to catch the last bus back to the nurses' dorm where I lived.

I had never failed to be impressed by the magic of Edinburgh. Somehow there had been a romance about the old grey city. Was it the floodlit castle standing majestically over me as I ran clutching my violin? Or the lights of Princes Street, dissipating to the little stables behind the castle? Or was it something deep within me, an affinity with my ancestors who were so proud of our Scottish heritage?

Whatever it was, it excited me as much now as in those orchestral days. Edinburgh had become home to me in so many ways: my first home after leaving the family nest in Birkenhead; the place of my nursing and my friends; my first years of marriage to Matthew. It had embodied my life, and I loved it.

It had also, of course, been the place where I had first become ill after an appendix operation eleven years earlier. It had been a desperate illness which had changed the course of my life. Yet that memory, though full of anguish, neither spoiled nor tainted my memories of Edinburgh itself.

Now, ten years after leaving, we had returned again for a week—a welcome few days in which to catch up with old friends and old vistas.

Matthew carried on reading the front of his newspaper while I approached, slightly breathless from running. He was quite unperturbed by my being late.

"Sorry I'm late," I stuttered when I got my breath back. Then, eagerly, "I met Jocelyn."

He folded his paper slowly, still reading the end of his paragraph. "That's fine," he replied distantly.

It was never a good moment to tell him anything when he was reading.

"No, it's not fine. It's surprising," I pestered.

Matthew stuffed his paper down the side of my shopping bag. "Start again," he invited, reluctantly.

I was impatient with myself for dragging him out of his enjoyable reverie when I could have waited. Perhaps it wasn't so important anyway—although, somehow, I could not get the thought of Jocelyn out of my mind.

"Jocelyn," I began again to Matthew, slipping my hand into his as we started up the hill. "We had a chat. A good chat. She seemed amazingly open."

"Good," came the reply.

"I got the feeling that there's an awful lot more to her than we ever knew while we lived so near to her in Edinburgh."

"Mmmm," Matthew was still slightly distant. "There is."

We were about halfway up The Mound now and stopped to admire the view. Together, we peered through the spiked iron railings, grasping their cold rustiness in both hands as we gazed toward the pinnacles of the Walter Scott monument. Silently we each cherished our memories of the place.

"Do you remember that day we were going to meet for lunch at the domestic science college, and I was terribly late?" Matthew mused.

I remembered particularly clearly. It had been immensely embarrassing, since we had been invited as guests of a staff member at the college. A special lunch had been presented that day because the students were being examined for their diplomas. Matthew and I had kept everyone waiting—examiners, staff and students—for half an hour.

"Yes," I replied, trying to quell the old resentment I had felt when he had been so late.

"Well, that day . . . " he smiled philosophically as he recalled the whole situation, "I was late because of Jocelyn. I couldn't just get up and walk off from all that she was saying. It proved to me beyond any doubt that you never know what lies concealed inside people."

He drew back from his stance of leaning against the railings and we set off once again. "You never know . . . " he repeated.

I swallowed hard. Not only had I been unfair to Matthew, blaming him for being so late, but also to Jocelyn. I had been so busy pitying myself, it had not occurred to me that she had needed to talk that day—even if that meant delaying Matthew and the students. Whatever she had said, it had been really important to her. I had not known from Matthew. He never talked to me of other people's confidences. Only occasionally, as now, he gave little clues. And I had not guessed. She always looked so composed, so much in control. I could have used Jocelyn's own words: "I just never knew . . . "

In silence together, we walked on toward the castle at the start of our autumn vacation.

2

Stone or Bread?

*Which of you, if his son asks for bread,
will give him a stone? (Matthew 7:9)*

It was a good vacation. Most of the week we spent with friends in Fort William, going out each day to drink in a different view from the surrounding hills or glens. Until one morning, we were able to disregard the burden imposed by my physical limitations.

On that day—our last before returning to Edinburgh—we awoke to sunshine streaming through the yellow curtains of our bedroom. Pulling them back, we looked out to see the first sprinklings of snow on Ben Nevis, sharply etched against the clear blue sky. Without wasting any more of such a perfect day, we decided to set off for the west coast toward Mallaig.

Matthew packed the car while I gave the children a quick breakfast. They shared our high spirits. Philippa squealed with delight in typical two-year-old fashion while Angus fidgeted excitedly on the bench where he sat eating his oatmeal. "We're going to the seaside!" he sang. That was more interesting to him than any spectacular views *en route*—even when they were enhanced by the rich colors of the autumn.

Then came the blow. It was like a thud which, as it hit me, knocked me off balance and spun me around. Excitement was turned to something solemn; pleasure was tainted with grief.

I had noticed Matthew rechecking his hiking boots at the car. Now, as I cleared the table, he came in and laid the map on the crumby surface.

"How would it be if I were to do a climb on my own, lady?"

Thankful that I had not made some churlish criticism about putting a clean map on the crumbs, I bit my lip. This was a precious holiday; each day was to be enjoyed.

"Oh?" I gave a neutral response, allowing time for the rush of negative reactions to slow down.

It wasn't that I resented his going. The weather was perfect. The views would be wonderful. And whereas he usually went on many hikes, this week he had so far done none. This was his last chance.

Nor was he avoiding time with the family. He had given so much of his time for us. Each day he had taken the children in turn down the long water slide at the swimming pool, giggling wildly as they belly-flopped off the end. Whenever we had stopped beside a loch or river, he had not just watched passively as they threw stones into the water, but he had joined in, enthralling them by the splashes he created as he tossed huge boulders. At the end of each afternoon he had read stories by the log fire in traditional, fatherly manner with the two children snuggled on either side of him. He had thus also created welcome space for me to read or rest quietly on my own for a change, without being climbed on or poked. It had been marvelous.

"That would be nice for you," I tried not to emphasize the last two words. To have done so would have burdened him with what was my own problem.

"I thought I'd do my favorite walk up . . . " he pointed to the brown area on the map where the contour lines hugged one another closely, indicating an interesting ridge, "here."

I dried my hands and looked. *Creag Bhan.* I had thought so.

"Isn't that where there's a funny wooden bridge by the roadside?"

"That's right." Matthew did not ask how I remembered it so clearly. "I'll take this path, here." He traced the dotted black line which indicated the narrow path.

I knew that path. It was the one on which I had tried to climb a mere 1,600 feet, but had not managed it. I had not gotten past the lower slopes to which Matthew's forefinger was pointing. It had beaten me.

That walk represented to me what might have been. We had done so many walks together in Scotland. Until my third operation, hiking had been one of our special pleasures—something which strengthened the bonds between us, helping us to feel close to one another. If only I had not been so ill, for so long, we might have been climbing together today.

I looked at Matthew's strong frame bent eagerly over the map. I wanted to say, "It's not fair! I want to come too." If only I had been better, and stronger, it would have been possible. Philippa could have been carried in the toddler backpack and, although he was only five years old, Angus could have walked it. He longed to join such adventures.

But there was no question of my doing it. It had been only ten days since I had emerged from the anguish of yet another two months of more abdominal infection . . . only a fortnight since the doctor had been administering strong injections to help me through a particularly bad night of pain. To have travelled so far at all was surprisingly good; to go gallivanting on the hills would have been folly.

I struggled to quell my self-pity. "That's fine," I said, trying to sound sincere. I hurried to bundle us all into the car. Then, at least, my face would not be seen.

"I hope you really enjoy it," I tried to sound enthusiastic for Matthew as he laced up his boots by the bridge. "You should be able to see Skye and the Cuillins as well today." My words were sincere, but I knew my eyes did not sparkle as if I had been seeing them for myself. How I wanted to see our honeymoon isle from that peaceful hilltop!

Angus, Philippa and I waited and waved until the figure of Matthew had become a small orange dot progressing up the hillside, and then we headed toward Arisaig. It was a beautiful drive. The route swept through gorges and glens lined by the rich colors of the autumn. Larch trees stood tall and stiff like a guard of honor; beeches hung their lower branches to the ground like men holding their caps in a sweeping bow of salute; glades were carpeted by leaves like garlands of flowers strewn along our way.

But only half of me was there. The other half had set off with Matthew. I could envision him now ... He would be up by the hidden loch—Loch Beoraid—where the path forked. I had seen some deer there on the day I had attempted the walk alone. I had come upon them quite unexpectedly, standing stock still as if they had been waiting for me to emerge over the brow. We had stared at each other for a moment, then, at the stag's lead, they had all fled down into the glen.

I had stood gazing down at their tiny brown figures, almost invisible now, as they gathered once again into the coziness of the herd. Only my breathing had broken the stillness. Puffing already from exhaustion, I saw the white coils of my own breath curl upwards. I had been prepared to relish the magic of the moment until, perching on a boulder, I had become aware of the hammering thud of my heartbeat.

It was then that I had no longer been able to see the view. A darkness had imposed itself heavily over my head and my eyes like an ominous cloud. Then it had pressed in on me, pushing me down, down, down. On all sides I had felt pressed and squeezed, accompanied by that dreadful, crescendoing, rhythmic banging noise which was no longer a muted thud. It had grown into a metallic din which threatened to bulldoze me any moment.

For a second I had sat paralyzed, engulfed in

confusion, aware of my limbs trembling while nausea swept over me. Quickly I had lain down; I did not know for how long. Gradually the pressure had eased, the darkness lifted. But of course, I could not have gone on.

It had been a terrible moment. I had never dared to tell Matthew the full horror of the darkness. "I got a bit tired, so I didn't make it to the top," I had said. Was it fear of looking stupid which caused me to underplay everything? Did I make myself sound more strong by saying "a bit"? Or was I just trying to avoid dramatic exaggeration—a trait from my family which was a great source of amusement and mockery, even amongst ourselves.

Whatever the case, Matthew had been very kind. "Never mind," he had assured me. "Another time, when you're fitter, you'll make it to the top. On a clear day, there's a stupendous view."

He would be about halfway up by now.

The Mallaig road curved its way toward the sea. A truck was approaching our car. I had become so caught up in thinking of Matthew and in reliving my own walk that I had not noticed the road had narrowed to only a single lane. Suddenly I had to jerk the steering-wheel sharply to pull into a passing place. The tires skidded on the loose gravel at the side of the road as I swerved and shuddered to an undignified halt.

The driver of the truck glowered from behind his gold-rimmed spectacles. I tried to appear unflustered as he passed, giving a gracious wave and smiling reassuringly to him as if I had been in full control of that skid. His face remained set and dour. He was unconvinced.

"That was a close one, Mommy!" came a voice from the back.

"That close one!" echoed Philippa, aware that something exciting had just happened.

I prickled uncomfortably. I did not like to be corrected, especially by the children. And I was a little too shaken to be able to laugh at myself with them.

"Look at the lovely colors," I suggested, trying to avoid the subject. But Angus found it much more interesting to speculate about car crashes and relish the idea of the car nearly having had a big dent to show Daddy later, if only I had gone a bit faster.

I sat myself up straighter. I could not allow myself to lose my concentration. Arisaig would not be far off now. The dark woods had opened out and the road was no longer shrouded by trees.

"Let's have a picnic here," I suggested at last, drawing up beside a deserted white beach.

We piled out enthusiastically. The openness of the sparkling blue sea felt fresh and unoppressive. However beautiful the trees had been, it felt good to have come through the valley. We could anticipate a new sense of freedom.

"Big sandpit!" cried Philippa in utter delight as soon as she came upon the beach. Then she was stamping her feet and splashing the water's edge.

"Yes," I chuckled contentedly to myself, pleased to be pulled back to the freedom of a child's unfettered enjoyment. "And over there you'll find some shells to collect and stones to throw into the sea." I found a place for myself in the shelter of a large rock and spread out a blanket. That could become a home base for the next couple of hours.

The children raced off immediately, abandoning themselves to the freedom and space. They ran and they laughed, chasing and playing excitedly. The sun, beaming down on the sea, caused the water to dance and wink in sparkling delight with them. I relished its balmy warmth, despite the lateness of the season.

Soon Angus began a project, building channels in the sand for the water to run. Philippa, being younger, kept closer to me as she collected her shells and stones, bringing each one for me to admire before toddling off for more.

I thanked her dutifully for each item she placed into my hand before adding them to a pile. Mostly, they were small pebbles—until one stone.

"Bread," said Philippa, as she handed it to me. I smiled benignly, not really understanding her. "Bread," she said again.

Was she saying that she wanted some bread? Her vocabulary did not yet extend to verbs, but I knew it was almost lunchtime.

"That bread," she repeated. She pointed purposefully to the stone. I gazed at it, then back at her quizzically.

"That roll!" she explained so loudly that she was shouting in her endeavor to make me comprehend.

Suddenly, I saw. The stone was the shape of a bread roll, and she was sharing her observation.

"Oh, yes, Philippa!" I gave her a little hug. "That

is like bread. It's the same shape as a roll. Good girl!"

She toddled off once again, content to have gotten through to me at last. *How intriguing,* I thought as I watched her, *that she had seen the shape of a bread roll in a stone. She was so right.*

I held the smooth roundness of the stone, stroking it with my fingers. For a second, my forehead puckered. I had read about bread and stone together before. It was in the Bible. I knew the passage well: "Which of you, if his son asks for bread, will give him a stone?" (Matthew 7:9)

It was strange. Jesus also had been at a lakeside when He had spoken those words. I closed my eyes, smiling inwardly to see the parallel. Could Jesus have seen the same similarity as Philippa had and been holding a bread-shaped stone which He'd picked off the shore?

Philippa's stone lay cold, hard and heavy in my hand. It was very different from the soft feel of good bread. There was nothing nourishing, nothing good in a hard stone. I shuddered a little.

Jesus' words continued to ring round my head. He had been talking about prayer. He had compared nourishing bread with hard stone in order to show the goodness of God. He had been testifying to God's nature, that He always gives good things.

But the words unsettled me. They did not convey the warm reassurance that others seemed to find in them. Other people could say that God had never given a stone instead of bread. They implied that He gave them whatever good things they asked of Him.

My experience was different. The "bread" for

which I had asked was freedom from pain, and He had not given that. I had asked for a miracle of healing and I had not received it. Instead, I had been left with more pain, more infections, more operations. The cold, hard fact of that going on and on had seemed like receiving a heavy stone.

I put Philippa's stone down in the pile and sighed.

I did not understand. Why did God say in the Bible, "Ask and you will receive," when it was not always as easy as that?

I knew that God did not offer Himself to be used as the obedient genie from the story of Aladdin. Reluctantly, I had to accept that prayer was not a case of rubbing a lamp and calling for whimsical gifts by magic. To have tried to do so would put me in the position of God. He would have been subject to my orders. That made a mockery of God's sovereignty.

Sometimes, when I had been struggling with this, I had been told that the key was to ask "according to God's will." But surely, it must have been within His will to ask for healing. Yet here I was, eleven years later, unable to climb a hill with Matthew because of the persistent abdominal pain.

I leaned forward and fiddled distractedly with the stones, flicking them up in the air and catching them again before tossing them crossly back into their pile. But I could not toss that verse out of my mind: "Which of you, if his son asks for bread, will give him a stone?"

I did not believe that God dangled carrots of hope in a taunting way. I trusted Him to fulfill all His promises. However much His answer to my prayers seemed like a stone, instead of bread, I could not believe that His words were untrue. So what had Jesus meant?

The children ran over to the blanket. "Come on!" I invited them. "Who's ready for our picnic?" I gathered up Philippa's stones and stuffed them into my pocket. We had to keep them. They had become her treasures.

With hands outstretched, they reached for their rolls. Philippa made no comment about her stone. We all took and ate.

We were quiet, relishing the tranquillity and the sea. The children, exhausted from their energetic hours in the fresh air, were ready to sit beside me contentedly after lunch. Angus was very thoughtful.

"When I'm nine can I go with Daddy?" he speculated.

"Yes, I should think you'll be big enough by then," I replied. I stopped myself from adding wistfully, "If you're strong and healthy." I tried never to quench the bubbling spirit of fun and anticipation such as Angus was relishing now. Yet I realized that it was not a right that he should be fit and able to climb mountains. It was a gift and a privilege. My illness made me acutely aware of that.

My illness . . . It had taken over so much in the eleven years since the first simple operation. And whenever it threatened to dominate again, self-pity lurked just around the corner.

I leaned back on the blanket and sighed. I must try to relate to my own situation any philosophies I had about Angus. It was not a right for me to climb today with Matthew. It would have been nice, that was all. Why did I have to wrestle with myself so much in order to see it like that?

We lay back to rest on the sand. The bread-roll shape in my pocket jutted uncomfortably into my thigh.

♦ 3 ♦

Heart Broken

Sorrow, like a sharp sword, will break your heart
(Luke 2:35, GNB).

"But *how*, Jane?" Sarah's dark hair curled neatly over her shoulders, gleaming in the reflection of the log fire which crackled merrily in the grate. "How can we have courage when God seems to be asking intolerably painful things?"

I hesitated. I feared giving insensitive "answers" to what was painful for Sarah. She had every reason to talk about needing courage. All evening my eye had been drawn to the infant seat, poignantly vacant in the corner by the window. It was the one Sarah had used to lay each of her babies in after they had drifted off to sleep in her arms.

Matthew and I were spending the night at Colin and Sarah's home on our way south from where we had vacationed. Having bidden farewell to the Highlands, we had only the special anniversary party to look forward to before driving back to Cheshire. As soon as the children had been safely tucked in bed, the men disappeared to admire Colin's new computer, while Sarah and I had slipped into an unexpectedly deep conversation.

On the solid wooden sideboard at the far end of the room stood some photographs of their family. The children were a prominent part of their lives. But the beaming little baby framed by the most elegant silver frame caused my heart to be heavy. Robert's bubbling little life had been snuffed out.

Two years previously their unfettered joy had been shattered. Robert had become dangerously ill. His life had been threatened by a bleeding disorder. Everything had happened so quickly. What had started as an ordinary visit to the family doctor had ended with Sarah and her longed-for baby hurtling by ambulance down the street toward the hospital.

She had felt utterly bemused and disoriented. For hours, which had smudged into bleary days, she was mesmerized, engulfed in fear at what had been going on. But the medical treatment was to no avail. Before her horrified eyes, Robert's life was ebbing away. Within two days he had died. He was just eleven weeks old.

The following day had been a Sunday. Mother's Day.

Colin and Sarah had felt wounded and hollow, as if struck by a stone. Afraid of being told not to grieve, or to be thankful for the children who remained, they had not wanted to face visitors. The burial had been simple, and only snowdrops marked his little grave.

What could I say now to Sarah without trampling inappropriately on her feelings? There were no answers. Instead I turned the question back to Sarah herself, "How did you manage to have courage two years ago?"

She shook her head. "I found it so hard." Her eyes were sorrowful and heavy, and she spoke her words in spurts. "God seemed to be asking too much of me. He seemed to want intolerably painful things for me—that's why it was so hard to trust Him!" She glanced up to check my face, lest she had shocked me, but I was nodding silently. In my limited experience I had felt that sort of fear, too.

"I was afraid that He might dismiss my feelings in place of His own, which made me feel desperately alone," Sarah explained.

"So how did you manage to get through?" I asked gently.

Sarah closed her eyes against the painful memory. "It all seemed such a waste, so futile. I was angry at the idea of having to go through with it. Angry in case God thought it was 'good for me' or something." Her voice trailed off for a few seconds. "But among all my anger at God there was a question. It kept repeating itself with stark simplicity: 'Do you believe in the goodness of God?' "

I was silent, intent as Sarah bared her soul. "One night beside Robert's empty crib," she said, "I remember looking helplessly in it, weeping and sobbing. I felt as if I'd reached rock bottom. I cried out, 'Lord, please don't ask me to go through Robert's death!' His only response was the constant repetition of the question, 'Do you believe in the goodness of God?' "

Sarah's eyes were brimming with tears once again as she recalled that night. "Somewhere . . . somewhere among all my fear, I was aware of a flicker of hope. I knew it had to be a lie to imagine that God would impose dreadful things on me, disregarding how that seemed to me. That was like the glimmering light of dawn. I had to concede that His purposes are for good and not for evil."

I pressed my lips together tightly as I listened. I was inspired but also strongly challenged. How would I have responded if faced with the same question as Sarah? I shuddered to think of having to bear loss such as hers. Would I have found the same peace? I might have shared her doubts, that God had taken her further than she felt able to endure. But her faith seemed so strong, resisting the lure to believe that God had let her down.

Did I believe in the goodness of God as Sarah did?

Sarah must have read my thoughts. "Don't get me wrong. It was desperately hard," she tried to explain.

I took up her cue. "As if God were giving you a stone . . . " I suggested pensively.

"That's right," Sarah agreed. Her voice sounded grateful that she did not have to convince me further.

"As if He gave a stone when you had wanted bread. You had even prayed for bread." My thoughts were miles away as I spoke. "And instead you felt God was asking you to accept Robert's death . . . " I sensed again the discomfort of that stone jutting into my thigh at Arisaig. I looked up questioningly.

"It must have seemed as if God gave it without caring too much about how hard it was . . . "

"Yes!" Sarah exclaimed, surprised at my directness. She seemed to relax a little at the relief of being allowed to be honest.

"But when you yielded to Him?" I asked her.

"Jane, the only peaceful course for me was to trust in His goodness." She shrugged, bewildered at the paradox. "I suppose the big question is about prayer. Does God have His own way anyway? Does it matter what we ask Him to do?"

I sighed, discomforted again. Sarah sat up straighter. "Jane, I asked you this earlier. How do you pray when God seems to be asking intolerably painful things of you?"

I leaned my elbow on the arm of my chair and rested my chin on one hand. The flames in the fireplace licked around the chunks of wood like forked tongues. One log slipped down with a raw, scraping noise and nestled more closely into the grate.

"I never pray in only one way," I began. "And undoubtedly, it is a struggle, Sarah. Sometimes I don't want to speak to God at all."

"That's it," she jumped in quickly. "That's what I'm asking. How do you pray when God seems not to care about how black life is?"

For some moments I reflected. I closed my eyes and pictured the little corner which I set aside for praying.

"Someone once sent me a card with a prayer by St. Thomas More," I finally said. "That card both challenged and comforted me. I stuck it on the wall of my study, where it faces me whenever I kneel to pray. It reads, 'Thank you, Lord Jesus, for what you have given me, for what you have taken away from me, for what you have left me.' "

I paused before confiding, "It's taken me years to be able to make that my real prayer, instead of just saying the words."

My forefinger traced the leafy patterns on the arm of my chair. I was struggling to be honest. It would have been much easier to have sounded confident, as if such godly prayers came easily to me. "Even now I can hardly bring myself to mean it. I need God's healing hand all the time to help me in that."

I looked up at Sarah sitting with her feet tucked up on the seat of her chair. Her face registered surprise, even bewilderment. She had imagined that it was only she who lacked courage when faced with suffering, and that I sailed along spiritually without a hitch.

"It's much easier to use those words to accuse God for all that He has not done for me," I began. Behind Sarah's puzzled expression there was a glint of understanding. She waited for me to explain.

"When I start reading the first line, I try to think of the many pleasures and fulfillments God has given me. But even before I have time to focus on them, I spoil it. Thoughts rush into my mind as to what He hasn't given me. My imagination runs wild. Almost instantly a whole list of items parades before me. And so, instead of uttering the words themselves, I find myself wanting to pray, 'Lord, how can I thank You for what You have given me, when You seem to have overlooked other really important things . . . like health and strength and stamina?' "

Sarah shuffled a little in her chair.

"I hurry on to the second line, 'For what You have taken away from me.' I hardly dare say to you, of all people, how hard it is to thank God for what He's taken away. My own mind invariably flits to what has been taken away surgically at each abdominal operation. Again, I want to say to God, 'How can I thank You for all that has been taken away? You've allowed more to be taken away than I can bear!' "

Sarah's face urged me to continue.

"But up on the wall in front of me, the words on the card do not change. They just sit there, so unchanging they seem almost stubborn. And all the time that I think of things which He fails to give me, they seem to stare back at me as an uncompromising reproach. I suppose it must be a bit like the question repeating itself in your mind, 'Do you believe in the goodness of God?' In the end I have to bow to them and to the Lord. I kneel before Him and I speak the words of that prayer. It is in speaking them that I find a sincerity and conviction almost as strong as my initial excuses not to say them at all."

I paused for a moment, picking distractedly at a loose thread on the armchair, twisting it between my fingers and poking it through to the reverse side.

"Then I reach the last line." I was unsure how honest I wanted to be. Haltingly I went on, "By then, I feel humbled. That in itself must be God's graciousness in hearing my prayer. Yet, somehow, that's the line over which I most want to shout at God."

I fell silent, deciding not to reveal all my resentments which seemed shamefully petty in comparison with Sarah's grief.

"Please, tell me why?" Sarah prompted gently. The warmth of her voice encouraged me a little, reassuring me that she would not despise me for sharing my feelings with her. Far from being either appalled or even bored, as I had feared, she was actually able to see them as a part of my pilgrimage with God.

I glanced up at her. It was my turn to confirm that I could trust my friend. "Those words evoke thoughts yet again about my operations. It's just so easy to slip into bitterness and stop thanking God for things! I find myself accusing God, 'But I wasn't left with anything!' The operation in 1980 was a total pelvic clearance. Nothing was left." My fingers tightened tensely into my palm.

Sarah was puzzled. "Why is that so significant to you, Janey?" she pressed gently.

"Because that represented a threat to the whole of my womanhood. My ovaries were only a small part of what was removed, but if even a tiny part of one ovary had been left, that would have been sufficient to control my hormones normally. As it is, though, it's only drugs which keep my blood levels — well, me — female."

"Couldn't they have thought of that?" Sarah tried to understand.

I grunted bitterly. "Oh, they tried. The surgeons performing the operation tried to be as conservative as possible. But they had no choice. My pelvis was so badly damaged by repeated infection that everything had to be removed."

Sarah nodded with understanding. She had

been closely involved with Matthew and myself during that most severe bout of peritonitis in 1980.

"It's okay," I shrugged, trying to resume my former casualness. "Mostly, I can laugh it off and join in with the jokes about female hormones. But sometimes I feel the hurt of that loss. Well," I flicked a white feather off the chair cover, "they're still an integral part of being a woman. Without them, it's as if I've been sort of neutered. It took months, if not years, before I brought myself to wear pants after that operation. I had to persuade myself that I was still feminine, even by the clothes I wore."

Sarah gazed toward me sympathetically. "I never realized," she said.

I blushed, suddenly ashamed to be receiving sympathy. "It's a private thing in our culture," I told myself more than Sarah. "Anyway," I tried to deflect the conversation away from such self-indulgence, "I can tell you, God certainly realizes. I tell Him often enough. Every time I pray that prayer, for example!"

We both giggled, and relief washed over me again.

"Do you ever pray the whole thing then, Janey?" Sarah pursued, after the laughter stopped.

"Well, amazingly, yes. I do. One of the things I've learned is that once I face up to things which hurt, they can actually become seeds: seeds for growth. I think I make a conscious effort to switch my mind away from wallowing around in the same old story. After all, Thomas More can hardly have been thinking about abdominal operations when he wrote that prayer! Remembering that helps me to set my mind on more spiritual things."

"Like what?"

"Well, things like faith I suppose. I mean, He's never taken that away, no matter what has happened. But then, I've not had to face pain such as yours . . . "

I swallowed, shivering once more just imagining Sarah's mourning. "Sarah, you know this too. It's faith which tells you — and me — that God is good, no matter what we feel. He is a loving Father. We can trust Him that He won't give a stone when we ask for bread. Though, I admit, sometimes it takes courage to cling on to such a promise!"

Sarah interrupted, "But Jane, I don't think I've that courage at the moment."

I pursed my lips. I knew that any courage was not mine, and it would only hinder her to think it was. Any faithfulness of mine was part of God's fruit, His harvest, born out of a struggle through pain.

"The only way I can pray that prayer is by remembering who God is. If He's in charge of my life, then He's in charge of every detail — including what happens at the hand of surgeons while I'm asleep. I have put myself into His hands. Nothing can be done by anyone, except under His guiding hands. Nothing has been taken away without His permission. I don't understand His purposes, but I trust Him. Only in that way can I blurt out my thanks to Him, silently asking Him to accept my hesitancy, too." I paused, then added with a smile, "He always does."

Sarah's admiring gaze rested on me.

"I don't want you to think that I am full of trust and courage," I quickly said. "It's God you must admire, not me. It's His harvest which I am amazed to be discovering. I just come upon it, springing up unexpectedly. So I know He is in it with me."

Sarah was still waiting for me to say more.

"When something dreadful happens, we start off resenting it, or wondering how on earth God can allow such suffering. We can only see it in terms of ourselves and the distress it causes to us."

Sarah nodded.

"But after a while, when we stop shouting at the air or asking other people why—in the end, when we ask God 'Why?' it's my experience that we have the joy of actually meeting God Himself."

Sarah raised her eyebrows before asking softly, "Have you ever met Him, Janey?"

I sighed impatiently. "Of course, I've met Him, and so have you. That change you just described that happened in you when Robert died, that was evidence of you meeting Him."

Sarah would never settle for less than the answer she sought. "I meant, *really* met Him?"

A puzzled frown crept across my face. "You know, there was an amazing thing which happened in Beverley . . . " I replied at last. My words came slowly as I turned things over in my mind.

"So what happened?" Sarah prodded gently. And I ventured to tell her.

◆ 4 ◆

Living Bread

Why are you talking about having no bread?
Do you still not see or understand?
Are your hearts hardened? (Mark 8:17)

January 1983. In the little hospital in Beverley I had to face yet another major operation.

It was one too many. For seven years, I had been succumbing to recurrent bouts of peritonitis. Some such infections had been so very severe that the inside of my abdomen was particularly messy. Each time, the doctors had used surgery in their endeavor to excise the seat of infection. They had taken out more and more until, in 1980, I had had what was called a "total pelvic clearance." That particular operation had been so drastic, its only consolation was that it should herald the end of my abdominal problems. Then suddenly, three years later, there I was again being prepared for surgery.

Perhaps it was the sense of let-down which was

the most difficult for me. Certainly my life had been saved in 1980, and I had been very much better through the following three years. But I had not been completely cured. Because the inflammation had never been eradicated, it still flared up angrily for weeks or sometimes months at a time.

Moreover, the surgery to drain such abscesses had been so extensive and difficult that it had left thick bands of scars—known as adhesions—between internal organs. These adhesions always pulled uncomfortably, but occasionally they also caused a twist in my gut—as in Beverley. The normal passage of food was suddenly obstructed. My whole abdomen was acutely inflamed.

I was cornered. There was no choice. I just had to go through with it. In the middle of the night I was rushed to the hospital and thrust once again through the whole business I knew so well. By morning it was evident that, without another operation to free the adhesions, the situation could quickly prove fatal.

The nurses finished preparing me for surgery and could check me off their list. They opened the curtains around my bed.

And at that moment I felt terribly alone. I was expected to face the world and cope, but I felt I could not. I could not muster up courage and be brave. I had none left. I could not face being so ill again.

A lady in the bed beside me looked across at me. Seeing the tears falling silently down my cheeks she must have concluded that I was just nervous about the operation. If only she had known . . .

"Poor dear," she muttered to her neighbor in a voice as near to a whisper as old ladies seem to manage. "She's young to be having all this done to her."

But that was not it. It was not my young age that made it so hard. I could have explained, had I had the inclination, that I had had more—much more!—than this at a "young" age. But what was the point? Could those alongside me ever have understood all about me? My history? Of course not. To expect that would have been unrealistic and selfish. As I knew so little of them and the hidden pain they faced, so too they had no indication of what lay behind my anguish.

No. It was not my age that I could not bear, nor even our human inability to understand one another fully. It was the relentlessness of the whole situation, the fact that my illness just kept on and on with its apparently futile course.

It was all so fruitless. Here I was facing yet another major operation, with the weakness and gaping loss of strength for months to follow, and for what purpose? Surely, if there had been lessons to learn, I had learned them by now.

Overwhelmed by the futility of it all, I buried my head under the starched hospital sheet. With a surge of panic I could only consider ripping out all the tubes and running away.

"No, Lord. I can't. I can't. I CAN'T!" I wept with bitterness.

At that very second Matthew walked through the door. His time as a minister was flexible, allowing him to drop in to see me whenever he chose. His face was calm and his eyes warmly loving.

"Matthew, I can't have another operation," I

blurted out before he had even reached my bed. He came over and lifted my limp hand into both of his.

"I can't face it. Not another."

"I know." His eyes showed little expression behind his glasses.

"No, Matthew. Don't you understand? It's more than I can bear."

He did understand. It was more than he could bear, too, to watch me suffer. But he didn't think of the hurt to himself then. He just looked at me kindly and repeated, "I know."

Perhaps his caring touch stemmed the flow of my torrent of panic and kicks. He said, "Let's pray." And before I could argue he had begun, asking God to be with me, to be beside me, to comfort me.

In the midst of my mundane and human panic in that awful hour, I was slow to acknowledge any answer to Matthew's prayer. Somehow I had found composure enough to go through with the inevitable surgery. But such was my desperation that, for a while, I was completely taken up fighting the battles within me that amounted almost to war. It took me some time to register also the peace which grew from that very fight.

About four or five nights after the operation, I was unable to sleep. I was at the awful in-between stage, knowing that I had improved because I had been promoted from an intensive care bed to a position halfway down the ward. The operation had been a success and I was certainly out of danger. But I was not yet better enough to be comfortable.

As I lay alone, I felt ill at ease. I tossed restlessly

in the bed, trying to sleep first in one position on my side and then another on my back. I longed to enjoy the release brought by sleep.

For five days, I had missed a special time of prayer or even of being still before God. Was that why I could not sleep now? I had to concede that I had no right to feel at peace in my soul.

Slightly guiltily, I tried to tune my thoughts into God's way of thinking. Still, I could not pray formally, but I was surprised to sense that God would accept even my most feeble attempts at thinking of Him.

Suddenly I was aware of God with me. There was no dramatic vision, but it was as if every cell in my body was being suffused with His peace. Whatever was happening to me, I knew it was God and that He was very big. He was so much bigger than I had imagined! Certainly this surpassed any human understanding.

My breath was almost taken away from me. Such closeness with God was all the more unexpected because I had not been in any specially pious attitude of prayer. Then He seemed to be calling me. His presence was so real that I was not surprised to hear Him use my name. It reminded me of the way in which the young boy, Samuel, had heard God calling him in the night. And so I wanted to reply to him, like Samuel. God's presence beside me was so near to something physical that I wanted to use my voice. Yet, aware of the other patients in the ward and not wanting them to overhear me, I merely whispered to Him, "Speak Lord, for your servant is listening."

God did not speak with an audible voice. But His Being was with me. Gradually, the special burning immanence of God began to fade. The whole experience felt so miraculous, I was sure there would be concrete evidence of having been visited by Him. He had been so close to me, it seemed only logical that there would be some physical sign of His powerful presence. My first thought was that my wound would not only be healed, but that there would be no wound at all. No scar. No stitches.

I slipped one hand under the covers of my bed. Gently, I began to peel back the bandage down one side. Gingerly, slowly, I eased my finger down the side of the dressing to feel for the familiar shape of the stitches. I swallowed. I could identify the dried blood caked all around.

Unwilling to believe what my fingertips told me, I lifted the blankets a few inches and peered through the darkness. The light was very subdued in the dim ward, but I had been awake for so long, my eyes were accustomed to the darkness. I opened the little slot of white dressing which I had loosened. My heart seemed to thud more loudly.

The stitches were there. Ugly, black and caked with blood. Pus still oozed from one edge. How could there be no miracle when God had been so close to me?

My puzzlement did not last for long because, still, the glow of God's presence continued to flow through me. My wound was unchanged, but I was not. I had an unquestioning certainty that, whatever God wanted me to do with my life or my body, He was with me. He was to be trusted.

When, at last, my mind began to absorb what had happened, I was sure I should write down the thoughts which came to me. It all felt terribly important. So, as discreetly as any patient in a large open ward can switch on her bedside lamp at 2 A.M. without disturbing anybody, I began to write.

I described two different images. In my mind I pictured first some young seedlings which had been growing quietly and hidden. The coverings which had protected them were being lifted off in order to make room for them to grow. They would become strong plants and burst forth into fruit.

I scribbled excitedly: "They are the seeds which have been hidden within me since the start of my illness seven years ago. The fruit is the harvest which God will bring from pain."

The second image was of a castle. In it were precious jewels and these had been barred up, securely guarded. Now the castle was to be opened. I could almost hear the groaning of the drawbridge wood and chains as the bridge went down. Such groaning was symbolic of my own groaning and cries against the pain that I had had to bear. But it was not without purpose. God's plan, it seemed, was to reveal what was precious to all who chose to see them.

That night I caught a glimpse of pain as part of a transformation into a jewel—a precious stone. It was similar to irritant gravel becoming a pearl in an oyster's eye.

"I know He will do this," I wrote, "but I do not know that I will see it." I could have had no idea, then, of how much I would need to hold on to that assurance. Buoyed up by the wonder of God with me I went on, "That is insignificant compared to the sure and certain knowledge that God knows what He is doing. My time here in the hospital is not futile."

During the following day, I was still bursting with joy. (As I write now, I think that that joy has never left me.) Eager to share it then with friends who had prayed so diligently for me over a period of years, I wrote to tell them of the night's experience.

"Why has it taken so long for me to see?" I asked myself in that letter. Excitedly I told them how I had sensed God visiting me the night before.

"Please don't get tripped up being sorry that all this has happened. I am convinced that we mustn't be disappointed in God for allowing suffering to go on and on." I was quite elated by the magnitude of my experience, so fresh in my mind. "Last night has made the unpleasantness of my suffering pale into insignificance. I can say that only because I'm so sure that, under His tending hand, new growth will spring up and burst forth into fruit."

Somehow, through perceiving God's presence to be so very great, I could accept that my suffering was not some terrible mistake. I began to accept it as from my loving Father. I began to look, not to the stone which I had to accept, but to the One who held out His hands to me. He it was who met me that night. He it is who is the Bread of Life.

Jesus had experienced feeding on His Father God when He had been surrounded by stones in the wilderness. So in my wilderness I found that I was "fed" simply because my heavenly Father was there with me. I could say with Job, "I have treasured the words of [God's] mouth more than my daily bread" (Job 23:12).

God had revealed His presence within suffering, and my fear of being given a stone had been quelled, at least for a time. He had shown Himself to be immeasurably great. I could not have wanted better assurance. However much my pain seemed out of control, He was in control. That was enough for me. We can believe in the goodness of God. Since that night, I have never had any doubt of that.

Of course, some people do not wish to hear of such conviction. Or if they do, they prefer to write it off as unrealistically victorious. They prefer to think of God only as the One who visibly heals, rather than One who also works more deeply in us.

If my scar had been healed that night, others could have seen clear evidence of God, and they could have shared my joy. But mine had been a private miracle. I had met with the Lord, and He had graciously imparted a great gift. Not healing, as I would have chosen. His gift was of Himself. He was with me through whatever turmoil I faced. He would never leave me. And that seemed to me an even greater miracle.

It may sound very lame, but sometimes I forget this. I see what is near me and not what is beyond. I see the stone of continued suffering. I need to learn how to look behind that. Only then do I see the hand which holds everything, the Person who is the Giver. Only then do I see that hand as hurt and bleeding. He is the God who feels pain.

In my humanness, I lose sight of God. I feel surrounded by stones in the wilderness and I lose sight of the Bread of Life. I prefer to be confined within myself, to be weighed down by stones. I prefer to seek the bread that looks and feels soft and palatable than to relish the food He lovingly offers. Frequently I do not understand the love behind what I see, and I prefer to shun the stones and accuse Him, "That's not loving. You can't be loving to offer me that!"

But that experience was not to satisfy me for the whole of my life. Jesus is Living Bread. He wants me to feed on Him every day. He told us to ask for "daily bread"—not for a ration which would last for a week, but for years. Too often I try to depend on yesterday's bread—last year's bread. But like the Israelites with the manna in their desert, if I try to feed on yesterday's bread I find that it has gone stale.

And I guess that I am not very different from everybody else. I can become so discouraged, so bowed down by the pain itself, that I am lured back into believing that suffering is worthless. But as God continually nurtures me with His constantly outstretched hand, He transforms me into someone whom He can draw to Himself. Then I will be able to reach out not only to His hand, but also His heart.

Such acceptance has only been born from struggle. Indeed, the struggle is as essential to peace as a chrysalis is to the birth of a butterfly. Just occasionally I wish I were one of those people who sails blissfully through life without any battles.

But do they?

Silence Broken

*If I speak, my pain is not relieved; and if I refrain,
it does not go away (Job 16:6).*

We were the last to arrive.

We had come straight from Colin and Sarah's on the west side of Scotland, and by the time we got there the room was already buzzing with people. Anna, looking up from the table where she stood serving food, replaced her spatula and with outstretched arms exclaimed, "It's Matthew and Jane!"

The hub of party noise was hushed for an instant as people looked to see who we were. Those who knew how far we had come joined in a congratulatory cheer. Others nodded politely in recognition of our entry but, not knowing who we were, turned back to their previous conversations.

"What a wonderful surprise to see you both!" Anna gave Matthew a huge hug. "Absolutely wonderful!" she said when my turn came. We beamed at the warmth of such a welcome.

"But I thought you were only in Edinburgh last weekend?" she puzzled. "Weren't you on vacation?" Then she turned to her husband and children and asked, "Did you know they were coming?" Their eyes twinkled in affirmation as they revelled in this added dimension of surprise on their parent's silver wedding anniversary.

"Oh, you're all terrible. But this is such a lovely surprise. Do come over." She put one arm around each of us, guiding us toward the buffet table filled with tempting delicacies. "Come!"

We felt like star guests at this special celebration. Anna took it upon herself to serve us with fresh salmon caught earlier in the day by a friend. The silver trim around my plate added a final touch of sparkle, framing the greens and reds, the yellows and pinks of the salads. On the table, more hot dishes cooked in wine steamed deliciously. My mouth watered.

I looked up to take in the scene. The room was long, its walls lined with Anna's collection of pictures, all hand-painted by local artists. Trailing plants hung from the high ceiling and from the open fireplace a huge floral arrangement burst forth, its amber colors mimicking flames. In the unexpected warmth of that September, a fire was not necessary. Indeed, with the coziness of the party, the French windows at the far end of the room had been opened to allow guests to spill out into the garden.

Making my way through the room, I stepped outside to find the fountain playing merrily, the water dancing as if joining in with the festivities. On the lawn, small tables had been laid with white cloths, each one brought alive by its own candle which flickered only gently in the balmy breeze. Paper lanterns had been made and planted at various points among the flowerbeds, and the glow from their candles cast a mellow light all around. They were so simple: just wire coathangers reshaped to act as a frame for the translucent, colored paper. The artistic talent of all the family had been used to create a truly magical party.

Matthew and I picked our way among the guests toward some friends we had known well in Edinburgh. Soon we were laughing with them, reminiscing over past years as we dove into our generous platefuls of food.

"Well, how are you then?" Duncan's strong Fife accent bellowed amicably from behind us, and I felt a hearty thump of greeting on my back.

Matthew stood up to greet him, bracing himself to receive the repeated pumping handshake for which Duncan was often imitated.

"We're fine. What about yourselves?" he rejoined. I, seeing the vice grip turn Matthew's fingers white, rose as demurely as I could, making every effort to appear too frail for such overen-thusiastic treatment.

"And how are you, sweetheart?" Duncan asked, landing a great smack of a kiss on my right cheek. He grasped my waist firmly and stood back a little, holding me at arm's length while he looked me up and down. "Lovely as ever, I see," he answered for himself.

"Flattery, flattery," I began, embarrassed.

"It'll get you everywhere, of course," Matthew

finished my sentence for me. Everyone laughed raucously.

We resumed our eating and began to talk again with those on either side of us. We spoke of our vacation, so fresh in our minds, and Matthew told other hill-lovers of the deer he had seen during his walk alone up Creag Bhan. That, for him, had been one of the highlights.

Hastily, I turned to Mary on my left, and asked her about herself. All too soon the conversation came back to me.

"But how are you really, Jane?" she asked very kindly.

"I'm okay, thank you," I replied, preferring to pay more attention to balancing the fish on my fork.

"Really?" she probed further, unwilling to let me off with a shallow answer. From the corner of my eye I could see others lean over to catch my reply.

I tried to say more. "We've had a good vacation and a lovely family time. I myself feel rested. I'm well . . . enjoying a good patch at the moment." I looked round the table, hoping that everyone would be satisfied with the fullness of my answer.

Duncan's face crinkled into a broad grin. "Aye," he winked, "but we'll never know whether we can trust how well you are. Your cheery face has led many of us astray!" He leaned forward, pointing his finger conspiratorially, "You see, we know now that there's more to you than meets the eye. We've read your book!"

He sat back in his rickety garden chair, clearly satisfied with his observation. More eyes turned toward me, expectantly. Some people laughed, enjoying his direct manner, even if it was a little brash. On my right, Matthew's conversation about his climb had developed into an animated argument over which of the Cuillins in Skye he could have identified from his vantage-point. He was engrossed. I was not going to be rescued. I had to stand up for myself. I placed my knife and fork down carefully on my plate.

"Look," I said to Duncan, confronting his pointed finger directly. "If you've read my book, you'll know that I am reticent to talk about how I am. Just because I've admitted that and even written about it doesn't mean that I've changed. My personality is still the same. Now, how about telling me about yourselves?"

A shadow crossed Mary's face, as if suddenly she understood what I was saying. But before she had even formulated her thoughts to say more, Duncan was laughing again.

"I tell you, we're all fine!" he said, sweeping his arm in a gesture to encompass everybody. "We're chugging along happily enough, but life's distinctly boring without the color you two bring to it!"

We giggled. The conversation changed, and presently I wandered back indoors in search of some dessert. A trio of musicians had assembled and were beginning to tune up. I was so absorbed in watching the cellist secure the point of his instrument that it did not matter to me who may have heard me exclaim with great thrill, "Oh, what a magical evening!"

It was not until I looked up from pouring cream over my dessert that I saw who had been standing next to me.

"Oh, Jocelyn!" I felt as if our friendship had grown past the formal greetings of the previous week.

I followed her to her place alone at a table outside. She seemed as eager as I to spend some time together.

From another table we heard a great guffaw of laughter. It was Matthew with Keith and Duncan.

"They're having fun," smiled Jocelyn rather primly. Perhaps their frivolity was rather coarse for her taste.

I gave a reserved smile. "I think so," I replied distantly. Jocelyn changed the subject, asking kindly about our week in the Highlands. At length she asked, "Are you troubled about something, Jane?"

I looked back at her thoughtfully and smiled at her perception. "Well . . . " I began. Jocelyn's expectant gaze pierced through me. She read me very well.

I plucked up my courage. "Well, so many people ask me nowadays, 'How are you, Jane?' expecting me to give an honest and full answer. But all they say of themselves is 'Oh, we're fine,' or 'We're okay, thanks.' That tells me nothing! Why should I always be the one who has to open up?"

Jocelyn held her eyes on me without a flicker. The irritation I felt was in contrast to her unfaltering persistence. I steadied my voice and reasoned, "I know my pain is more apparent than theirs, especially since the book, but," I looked up at her doubtfully, "I think that's used as an excuse."

"An excuse?" Jocelyn looked uncertain.

"Yes," I said, recalling Duncan's recent outburst. "An excuse for them to point the finger at me. They seem to think I'm different for finding it hard to talk about my pain. I think that's an escape for them. Their pain stays locked up while I am expected to reveal all."

Jocelyn wore a very distant look, and her eyes drooped sadly. I could see that she had thought a great deal about our previous discussion on the cobbled streets of the New Town. Her voice held regret when she spoke.

"You see, I could have done so much more," she said. "I could have helped. I think that's why your book made me feel, well, uncomfortable really, that I hadn't done more." She scraped the last dregs of cream from her plate and looked up at me. "But I tell myself not to be guilty, because I hadn't known."

I frowned. "I didn't write the book to make you feel guilty about me!"

"Maybe not, but . . . " She sounded pensive now and still sad. I leaned both my arms on the small table and, finding my hands beside the candle encircled by its floral posy, I began to press distractedly at the wax.

"You see," I continued, "although I'm better at the moment, pelvic inflammatory disease is an ongoing condition. So, the people who live near to us now—what can I say to them? How can they help? They are around, but they don't know what to do. I don't know! They don't know how to help me now anymore than you did while we were in Edinburgh."

Jocelyn pulled a starched white handkerchief from her pocket and wiped her shiny nose very precisely. "Things would have been different," she said.

I could see that there was little point in fighting. I changed tactics.

"Jocelyn, if my book meant anything, then you'll know it wasn't just about me. You don't need me back in Edinburgh in order for you to do things differently. You're surrounded by others who are in pain, crying silently and hoping that somebody will care enough to notice the little hints which show there's something wrong. All unable to say . . . "

"Why didn't you say?" she pursued yet again, this time rather sharply.

"I tried to find ways of saying . . . " I paused. "I gave clues." Still she seemed unconvinced. Again I hesitated. At last I ventured, "And your pain?" I spoke softly, feeling myself flush immediately at my forthrightness to her.

Jocelyn braced her shoulders stiffly, then raising herself like the true lady she was, she conceded almost in a whisper, "That's very true."

I decided to say nothing, waiting. She was lost in thought.

She took out her handkerchief once again, but she spent so long rearranging it in her hand that I wondered if she was going to blow her nose at all. I watched her, trying to be patient.

"Do you remember," she asked at last, "one time when Matthew came to see me and he was terribly late for lunch?"

I nodded silently.

"Do you know, that was the first time I had ever talked about all that with anyone?"

Her question was rhetorical, but I wanted to answer her that I didn't know. I wanted to hold her back, to put up my hand and say, "Stop, wait a minute! Matthew doesn't tell me confidential things." But it was too late. She had gone too far. Memories of whatever had happened were already welling up in her mind, bubbling up—with bitterness, I wondered?—and tumbling out like the water in the fountain beside us.

"Do you know, it's twenty years since that happened?" She was lost in thought now, staring vacantly ahead. She had dropped into a trance-like state, remembering . . . "Twenty years."

Again I opened my mouth to whisper, "But I never knew . . . " But to interrupt her seemed somehow inappropriate. She was looking at me again, her blue eyes sharp and piercing.

"And do you know, not a day goes by without my thinking about it?" Her eyes focused on me disarmingly. "Every day," she emphasized.

I was fumbling to know what I should say. "Do you?" I heard myself ask lamely.

Perhaps—silently I tried to reason with my rising sense of impotence—perhaps I did not need to identify her hurt. Jocelyn had reached the time to share a tiny corner of what hurt her. She most needed me to listen, to be as sensitive to her hidden pain as to the kind of hurt which is easily seen. I could not twist so tender a moment into an occasion for me to pry.

Jocelyn was gazing blankly toward the garden

pond again with its lush shrubbery rising like new life from its muddy bank in the floodlights.

"Neither Edna nor I have ever mentioned it to one another," she said, "even though we live under the same roof. I've never brought it up. It's a closed subject." Her lips tightened together again for a moment, before she reflected distantly, "And she must feel even more badly than I do, since it was she who was at the forefront of it all."

She raised her handkerchief to her face at last, rubbing her nose roughly as if to blot even her thoughts away.

At that moment, Anna strolled across toward our table. I cast my eyes down and fiddled with the unused cutlery to conceal my intense frustration that our intimacy should be interrupted at such a point.

"This looks like a cozy little conversation," Anna called across to us as she approached. She sounded almost envious. Perhaps she had become rather tired of the more superficial chats inevitable for a hostess. I closed my eyes and swallowed, knowing that we could do nothing other than welcome her to join us at her own party.

"How are you enjoying this spectacular party?" I asked as warmly as I could. Her eyes sparkled with delight. I began to get up and drag a chair nearer for her.

Anna gestured for us not to move. "I didn't want to interrupt anything . . . "

We paused. I dared not look to Jocelyn, whose silence felt extremely uncomfortable. Her torrent of words had suddenly stopped. She must have felt as if the bright beam of the pond's spotlight had intrusively swung round to focus on to that part of her which, previously, she had always kept so carefully and meticulously hidden.

Quickly, as if being open about everything, I answered, "We were just talking about my book."

Anna raised her eyebrows expectantly and her full skirt rippled as she tucked it underneath her neatly, settling herself into the chair. "Well actually," I grinned, "Jocelyn was laying into me for not moaning more about my pain."

Jocelyn pressed her lips more tightly together and shook her head, as if despairing of ever helping me to see things differently. I gave a slight giggle. Though I had rescued her from exposure, I had rather taken advantage of her vulnerable silence. But the slight smile at the edge of her mouth reassured me that she accepted even my mischievous manner.

I thought I had provoked Anna to take my side and was waiting smugly for some soothing words of comfort.

"It's incredible to me that you should ever hide how you are from doctors and friends, when you obviously experience so much pain," she declared.

I swallowed. It must have been because I had not expected such a reply that I jumped in so quickly with a retort.

"It's not incredible at all!" I said firmly. Then, wanting to swing the spotlight off myself again, I added even more provocatively, "Everybody does it!"

I laughed, trying to soften what I had said so quickly, but clearly Anna could feel the sting as my words hit her. I tried to explain more gently, "It shouldn't be incredible at all that I, too, don't want to parade what hurts. I mean, look at everyone here, chatting contentedly, having a most wonderful evening."

We looked over our shoulders to the main hub of the party. "So many have said, like you, that they can't understand why I don't say how ill I have been. But the irony is that those who accuse me of that are probably hiding just as much pain themselves, though not necessarily physical pain. I mean, I can't be the only person here tonight who is in pain."

Anna watched the dancers thoughtfully. It was a progressive dance, and at the change of partners people exchanged greetings or, occasionally, a kiss.

"You're right," she said wistfully. She slid her knees back around under the table. "Seeing Mary with Keith reminds me. Have you heard that her husband is asking for a divorce?"

I gasped with surprise. When we had known them, Mary and Bob had had a stable marriage—or so it had seemed.

"I'm sorry," Anna said gently. "I thought you would have been told."

I shook my head, still stunned. To think that I had sat next to Mary just half an hour earlier and had not known . . .

"We're surrounded by people with needs, with pain of their own who need help, but who are all pretending to cope, just like me," I said.

"What do you mean, pretending to cope?" Anna almost ridiculed the phrase. "Is it just a pretence? Are we seeing a mask when we admire you for coping so well?"

"At times," I said quickly. "Undoubtedly so." Then I sighed ruefully, pleased to be challenged for once by someone who knew me so well.

"Appearing to cope can be pretence, I suppose. It's a mask if I say I'm fine just because I don't like or don't trust the person who asks me. I'm sometimes aware that there are other, intangible, subconscious reasons I don't want to be helped by them." I held my breath, surprised at hearing myself being so brutally honest. "But I don't know. Is it a mask? Or is it being appropriate?"

"Sometimes it's appropriate to be silent about what hurts," Jocelyn had at last regained her inner poise to be able to contribute to the flow of conversation.

She gestured with another of those gracious waves of her arm, toward those talking animatedly beyond us. "But sometimes we make it difficult for others to come close. We feel we have to."

Anna placed her hands in her lap, adding to the image of correctness already portrayed by her straight back. "But everybody's different," she countered, trying to sound more at ease with the conversation than she looked. "I mean, any suffering I may have is nothing compared to yours, Jane."

"Nonsense!" I snorted. "Absolute nonsense! There's no hierarchy of pain. Any pain hurts."

Both Jocelyn and Anna were silenced, so I continued, "For example, let me tell you about one of the people who wrote to me recently. He 'only' had a virus, but it went on for weeks. When he got no better and the dreadful headaches refused to leave him, a black depression enveloped him. His pain, though supposedly so minor, led him to the same miserable feeling as mine, that he would be better off dead than being left living with that pain. In fact, amazingly, he also came to the same reassurance of God with him—even though he'd 'only' suffered a virus—which he found very thrilling."

"But that's wonderful, Jane!" Both Jocelyn and Anna nodded encouragingly toward me.

"Yes, I suppose it is. But what I'm trying to say is that it unsettled me that he thought his suffering was milder than mine. He felt he had no right to feel as grim as I did. That's not so. His pain hurt. Surely pain is what hurts us—whatever that is."

Jocelyn, who had been listening very carefully, said quietly, "Jane, you ought to be able to understand why he felt that he shouldn't compare himself with you, though. I mean, a virus is hardly the same as peritonitis." Her voice resounded with the authority of one with medical knowledge.

I chuckled, but Anna took the opportunity to come back to her original observation. "You see, Jane, sometimes you appear to be coping so well. Perhaps it goes against you. Even when you're really ill, somehow your face appears bright. After all, there must be times when you want to cry."

I glanced across to Jocelyn. "Yes, of course there are. And when there seems to be nobody alongside me—even on the other end of the phone—that makes me feel more miserable and disillusioned."

"So why do you do it?" Anna pressed yet again.

Jocelyn smiled a warm smile toward me. Might she have known the answer to that question?

"There have been times when you've asked how

I was and yes, occasionally I have heard myself say that I'm 'Fine thanks,' when I'm not. If I just feel weary or sick—well, everyone feels like that at times. I don't think I should mope about such commonplace things. That would be boring."

"But it isn't. Don't you see? You're saying the same as that man with the virus. 'My suffering doesn't warrant attention.' But you yourself said that it does. And others want to help. You mustn't keep us at arm's length because you feel you should cope."

She had won. Wearily, I conceded, "I should probably have said to you, 'Look, can you come around and take the children for half an hour so I can lie down until this dreadful nausea passes?' But I have not dared to impose on people in that way. Partly, I think, that's as it should be. It wouldn't be fair to make myself an intolerable burden on others, because they do have their own problems. Partly, I admit, my failure to ask for help stems from fear. I am afraid that others might get tired of me if I were to make too many demands of them. I could not bear that."

My voice trailed off. But footsteps behind caused me to turn around just in time to see Duncan. He was approaching with glee, as if to pounce on me, but as I grinned back he simply offered his hand.

"Come on, lass," he invited. "We'll show them how to dance!"

I felt a new lease of energy surge into me. I rose, leaving the horrified faces of Anna and Jocelyn behind me for a while.

♦ 6 ♦

Temptation (I): Hard Stones

*Tell these stones to become bread
(Matthew 4:3).*

At first I thought it was just the flu. Both Matthew and Angus were recovering from a few day's infection, so when I began to feel shivery and lethargic one Thursday evening, my reaction was to be resigned rather than surprised. It was my turn.

Though I tried to stop myself from speculating about possible complications, by Friday afternoon I was perturbed by the increase in pain. I was pushing myself more than usual to try to ignore the normal abdominal discomfort. The weekend was fast approaching. Ought I to get the doctor's perspective?

Matthew would not be home until late. My shoulders tensed with frustration. He was always a better judge than myself of when to keep plodding on with the pain and when to seek medical help.

And while usually his work as a minister was flexible, on that day there was no such perk.

I glanced at the clock. Four o'clock. I would have to leave soon to pick up Angus from school. The very idea of the half-mile walk to get him daunted me. Was that just laziness? Bless him, he was the youngest in school and would be tired after an especially long day. He had been with his class to a play. I wanted so much to be a good mother. Could I muster the extra patience he would need from me if his tiredness made him cranky?

My immediate response was no. It was hard enough just to look after Phillipa, who had been using all the energy of any two-year-old to investigate my kitchen cupboards. I was preparing in advance for a dinner party the following evening. She had revelled in the afternoon's cooking, weighing ingredients with me, grating cheese with me, tasting everything from potato peelings to raw garlic. At least she seemed to be content and free from the cloud which was hanging over me.

As I tidied up, I knew I was dragging one foot after another. I was stooping involuntarily because of the pain. Fear grew inside me. I could not be ill. I was needed at home.

My fear was not only for the family. It was for myself as well. What if this pain and sickness were a sign of another crisis developing? Pain and vomiting are the first signs of an obstruction such as I had had in Beverley. Even the fleeting idea crossing my mind brought with it a heavy dread.

"I'm sorry," said the health center's receptionist on the telephone when I inquired if I could see our doctor before the weekend. "There are no more appointments."

"I see," I replied blankly.

"Unless it's urgent. Is it?" she continued, trying to be helpful. That was exactly what I did not know! I could not decide for myself. Was this just a slight increase in the normal pain which I have learned to expect, or was it developing and needing urgent treatment?

"That's what I wanted the doctor to tell me," I tried to explain.

"Well, if it's urgent you can come down here and wait to see him. The doctor will always see emergencies." She was beginning to sound like an automatic answering machine. "But of course, you may have to wait a long time since you don't have an appointment."

Of course. I thanked her and replaced the receiver. I turned to Phillipa, now trying to fit a huge metal serving spoon into her tiny mouth. She would soon need her meal. And there would be Angus, too, wanting me to listen encouragingly to his excited account of the play. I could not take both of them down with me for an indefinitely boring wait at the doctor's office. In any case, Matthew's meal had to be ready so that he could eat promptly before his evening meeting. No, I would keep battling on, keep hoping that the pain would ease.

It did not occur to me to cancel our dinner guests. I could usually rise to such an occasion, refusing to be flattened by pain. That Saturday, however, I spent the evening lying restlessly upstairs or sitting in the bathroom waiting to be sick. I felt that that might relieve the discomfort. But such relief did not come.

By the Sunday I was worse. It was consoling

that the children were being looked after on an adventure with granny. I could give in to the pull of my body, succumbing to the desire to go to bed.

"I'll be thinking of you," I assured Matthew as he bent over to kiss my forehead on his way to church. He knew that my thoughts would be prayerful.

"Thanks, lady." The use of his endearment reaffirmed his loving thoughts for me, too. "It's always amazing how the services go really well when you're at home praying—though I wish you could come." The sincerity in his voice helped me to feel slightly less impotent in this passive position of illness which I loathed so much.

Alone in the house, time became a blur. I knew of little: only the radio's droning voice which I could not be bothered to switch off. Soon Matthew was home again, telling me of the service and then bringing me some lunch on a tray.

I held the plate of mince on my lap. Matthew watched me caringly as I stared at it, then raised my eyes to him and back down to the plate. Suddenly my spirits plummeted. I could not possibly eat.

Matthew saw in my face the whole significance of that moment. We both acknowledged where this episode of illness seemed to be leading. There was nothing to explain, nothing to say. Matthew could see how I was, and he shared my fear. He had watched this pathway through pain all too often. It was a well trodden way for us.

He took my hand in his and, kneeling beside my bed, kissed it tenderly. "Dear Jane, I'm sorry," he said lamely. "I'm so sorry . . . " His voice trailed away. Both of us felt our eyes prickle with tears we did not want to begin to shed. We still had to go through the mechanics of enduring whatever lay ahead.

The doctor came out in response to Matthew's phone call. The one consolation for our low spirits was that it was our own doctor on duty that Sunday. His understanding of my medical history brought a wisdom we valued greatly.

On his way out he turned to Matthew. He was unashamed to share his uncertainty as to whether this was an abscess caused by yet more infection or an obstruction caused by the adhesions. But he had left some medicines to see if they would help.

"If she gets any worse, or if you're not happy about her," he said kindly, "don't hesitate to let me know." He knew of my reticence to seek help.

I hated this. I hated being so passive as to be talked about. I much preferred to be in control of everything.

By 10:00 P.M. we did have to call him back.

"I'm afraid I'm going to have to do the dirty on you," he told me apologetically after examining me. I opened my eyes, previously closed to hide the distress I felt. I was unsure exactly what he meant.

His gaze remained steady and certain. "I'm going to have to put you into the hospital."

I had been in the hospital so many, many times, I wanted to resist it again unless it was absolutely essential. I should have trusted him more, knowing that that was one of his goals, too. He had always delayed admitting me until he had no choice.

"Why?" I asked. My question sounded clinically objective.

"I'm not sure exactly what is going on, and there's obviously something wrong. I wouldn't be happy leaving you as you are." His quiet reasoning helped to counter my rising fear and apprehension.

I began to argue, "But if I'm in the hospital, it's so much easier for them to operate on me again." My voice sounded rather like a child's now, but I could not help it. "Why can't I stay here and see if it develops?"

He smiled compassionately. "I think it's developed enough now, compared with this afternoon," he replied. "We need to do X-rays, and you need an I.V. and adequate pain relief." His gentle tact and measured judgment made it easier for me to see reason. He was right. I had to capitulate. I was pretty sore now, especially after being prodded.

Matthew set about packing some things together for me to take. Why was he so calm? I did not share his serenity. I may have stopped denying how I felt, but that had only given way to apprehension instead. I knew that I sounded blunt now in all that I said.

"Have I got everything you need?" Matthew asked, folding fresh nightgowns into a case for me. Those nightgowns: how very frequently they had come to the hospital with me! "Is there anything I may have forgotten?"

"Clean underwear!" I replied churlishly. "They're the most important thing in the hospital."

Otherwise I said nothing. What could I say? It had all been said before. I think I had been through almost every reaction. There was nothing new. I just had to go through the awful mechanics of it all.

The ambulance arrived as the doctor was finishing writing his letter to the hospital staff.

"I don't want an ambulance," I sulked. Matthew tried to be lighthearted, chuckling at the idea that at least the neighbors would have some scandal to talk about.

The doctor did not look up from his writing. "You can't go by car in the state you're in," came his soft reply.

"May I have a sip of water?"

Crisply laundered covers were being flicked over me and the nurse smoothed her stylish corner. I had been made into a patient. Tubes had been stuck into me, injections given to me. At last I was being settled into the ward.

"Sorry," she replied, but without any regret in her voice. "You're probably going to have surgery."

Surgery! Her words struck into me. I could hardly manipulate my dry tongue to question her more.

"What, tonight?" was all I could ask. It was the least of all my questions, but in the immediate wake of her bombshell I wasn't able to think quite straight.

The nurse looked me over as if I was stupid. "Yes," she said curtly. "Didn't you know?" And without waiting for a reply she left, the noisy clomp of her smart shoes receding to another part of the ward.

She could not have guessed the effect of her words on me. I could not face another operation. *Could not!* How many times had I been in surgery — twenty? As in Beverley, my mind raced ahead, as if flicking quickly through a series of photographs. But alone in the darkness, I relived the horror of each of those moments with a vividness that astonished me.

Already I could envision the simplistic explanations by nurses too caught up in routines to know either that I had endured this so often myself before, or that as a nursing sister I had been the one to teach nurses such as themselves to help other patients through similar times. And I could envision now the long road to recovery, the gaping loss of strength, the insidious lowering of spirits. In the silence of the dark ward, with only the steady drip of the intravenous infusion to distract me, I wanted to run away from such a possibility.

I tossed about restlessly in bed. There was nothing I could do. I was completely helpless, unable to take control of events happening to me. I felt utterly taken over. Bound and entwined by pain again, stuck in that bed if not by the pain itself then by the tubes attached to me. Perhaps it was only in the loneliness of the long night that I was forced to face up to my own reactions. The truth was that I could have screamed.

What was the point of this episode? Had I not learned the lessons God could have wanted to teach me? How could I bear more? The thought of the anesthetic alone filled me with horror. I recalled one time when I had woken up on the operating table to find myself being resuscitated. Those few minutes probably contained the most harrowing moments of my life. To face another operation now was to associate myself with that experience. I could not do it. Surely, I would not have to?

"I hate this!" I cried in the quietness of the dark ward. "I hate this, Lord!" I repeated, as if to prove to myself that it was God whom I was addressing.

The steady drip of the intravenous infusion continued its silent course. Still I was alone in my anguish.

Did it matter to God that I felt unable to face more surgery? I had always felt sure that His plans were for the best—better even than my own. But when I was at my lowest it seemed that He disregarded the wretchedness I felt.

Why did God not rescue me? It seemed, as so often before, that He was doing exactly the reverse. He was allowing my suffering to continue.

I stared up at the bag of fluid feeding into my arm. Vacantly I tried to read its black writing, but my eyes refused to focus. The injection had blurred my mind. Once more I felt taken over. Flattened.

I determined not to give in. I had to steel myself against self-pity. I told myself not to become despondent. But my resolve was pretty feeble and I decided to read one of the Psalms. Perhaps that would help me to be inspired by how other people, more godly than I, had prayed when faced with onslaughts such as my own tonight. Clumsily, with my arm now bandaged around its intravenous tube, I reached for my Bible and turned to Psalm 27.

"The Lord is my light and my salvation—whom shall I fear?" I gazed through this first verse. Certainly I wanted this to be true. I wanted God to be my light and salvation. I wanted to believe in the goodness of God. But at that moment, I had to be honest. My trust in the Lord did not put an end to my fear of what might happen to me that night. Nevertheless, I read on.

"When my enemies and my foes attack me, they will stumble and fall." If only God would give a big sweeping decree which would have put such an end to my enemies . . . the pain, the sickness, the loneliness of suffering without comfort. But He had not. He seemed instead to hang back. He did not intervene. And His silence was like a stone: hard, cold and unyielding. Did He realize how hard His silence seemed to be?

I contemplated that question. Of course, Jesus had once had to face hard stones. His first temptation had been to change hard stones into something nice to satisfy His own need. Stones into bread. He had had the power. He had been filled with power at His baptism immediately beforehand. The temptation must have been very strong. But He had resisted. He knew that such a temptation was misuse of His Father's power.

Was it wrong for me to want such a transformation from stones now? Resolutely I read on. "For in the day of trouble . . . He [God] will hide me in the shelter of His tabernacle." This was my "day of trouble"—and it had stretched to a night of trouble also. Would God not hide me in His shelter? Eleven painful years of chronic infection I had had, with crises at times so severe that I had been close to death. I was on the brink of such an episode yet again. Would God not protect me from another operation, from the wretchedness I felt?

Tears welled up in my distraught eyes: tears of

anguish and of anger, too. I wanted God to protect me from the agony and distress I felt I could endure no more. Desperately, I cried to Him, "God, I need You to hide me in Your shelter most of all at times like now!"

Through blurred and watery eyes I forced myself to read on. Surely I would find some promise which would be true for me. "He will set me high upon a rock . . . " Where was this rock? I imagined it to be some kind of safe place where I could stand and escape the assaults of pain which battered and bashed me from all sides. There was no such way out for me. I was forced to go through with this whole dreadful saga: this pain, this night, perhaps even yet another operation.

Was I supposed to be comforted to read of others being rescued by God when I was not? This Psalm was not helping me in the way I wanted. I was looking for comfort which it didn't give. I could not share the same pious words to God as this psalmist. I could not praise God for rescuing me from my enemies. I was all too aware that I had not been rescued from my circumstances: I was still left with these wretched pelvic infections to which I succumbed.

I pushed my Bible away from me, down on to my knees drawn up with pain. I began to feel rather cynical. I did not want promises which seemed unlikely to be fulfilled in me.

Any hopes I might secretly have had for a spectacular miracle that night were dwindling. They seemed only naive fantasies now—castles in the air which symbolized my failure to accept how physically disordered my body had become.

Yet something inside made me uncomfortable.

Despite my sulks, I felt compelled to persevere to the end of the Psalm. I picked up my Bible again. A little further down the page I saw, "One thing I asked of the Lord, this is what I seek: that I may dwell in the house of the Lord all the days of my life . . . "

My conscience was pricked. I had not asked Him for only "one thing." Uppermost in my mind on that night was that I was asking Him for more than that: to be freed from pain. I was not single-minded as my Lord desired.

I swallowed rather guiltily, but still the page gripped me. Despite myself, I read on. Only a few lines down the page, three words caught my eye: "Seek His face."

My guilt was compounded. Others, I remembered, had also been moved by the stark challenge of those words. That phrase, quite simply, summarized God's desire for me. It encapsulated very clearly why He had created me. It was His only demand of me, and I knew that I had failed Him.

Fiddling uncomfortably with my I.V. tube, I hardly dared to seek Him in prayer. I knew that when I sought Him I did so as much for what He could do for me as for who He was.

I sighed and looked back over my own years of suffering. God had not rescued me from my pain. Yet I could not deny that He had been with me through it all. He had never left me.

Could that have been what the psalmist meant at the beginning of his Psalm, I wondered? I glanced back to the beginning. "The Lord is my light and my salvation—whom shall I fear? The Lord is the stronghold of my life . . . "

Perhaps I could say the same. Without the

Lord, I would certainly have had no stronghold at all. I would have been utterly swamped. The horror of being told of this next possible operation could have grown into an all-consuming despair.

A flicker of new understanding dawned on me. *Despair.* Yes, I thought to myself, that's my real enemy. More than the abdominal pain which takes over my body, despair eats into my very soul.

I began to sense that this Psalm could relate to me after all. I looked back to the top of the page again: "When my enemies and my foes attack me, they will stumble and fall . . . Then my head will be exalted above the enemies who surround me."

My head had not been lifted above physical pain. But suddenly I saw that suffering was not my worst enemy. My enemies were those things which crept unseen into my soul and fed despair. They were the ugly things like self-pity, resentment, bitterness, pride. And God could lift my head above all of those. He could set me high upon a rock to shelter me from them. He could hide me in His shelter away from them. He does so whenever I seek His face.

Again I slid my Bible down to my knees, but this time not in anger. It was to allow myself to pursue what the Psalm had meant.

This was "a time to hate." Hating my pain was fruitless, disheartening and introspective. But hating my self-pity would sow seeds for the growth of love. What God wanted was for me to stop justifying my sins and to hate them.

My thoughts were interrupted by the arrival of the senior surgeon. Immediately any sense of peace gave way to a surge of panic. Once again I was questioned and prodded.

"Well?" I asked, watching his anxious expression. He moved toward the end of the bed and studied the charts hanging there.

"I'm not sure," he answered evasively. "My own instinct is to operate immediately." My pulse quickened. He seemed distracted, intense.

"However, I've just been speaking to your doctor. He knows about you better than I." He replaced the charts and looked at me doubtfully. "He says we're not to open you up tonight."

I felt myself breathe once more. Immediately, however, the next question was on my lips. "What then?"

The surgeon gathered the file of case notes together and dumped them on the bed-table. He edged away.

"We watch and wait," he answered, then disappeared.

7

Seeds Within Pain

It is the Father, living in me, who is doing His work (John 14:10).

There are seeds within pain—seeds which will eventually grow and yield a harvest.

At the time it doesn't feel like it. The seeds may not be visible. They may be too tiny. They may be hidden beneath the surface, just as any seeds need to be buried under the ground for a while.

Yet they are there. New seeds had been sown during that episode in the hospital—seeds not only in me but also in those close to me who suffered their own pain as a consequence of mine.

Both Matthew and I were probably the last ones to recognize such seeds. And we would not have appreciated being "encouraged" had such a suggestion been made. That would have seemed empty consolation. When seeds are sown in tears, the tears may be so all-consuming that they draw all attention away from any possible fruitful purpose.

For myself, newly home from the hospital, I was taken up with the everyday slog of just getting through each day, pushing myself on toward a fuller recovery. Matthew, on his part, could see nothing positive. The truth was, he felt utterly thwarted.

It was this feeling which was uppermost in his mind when he went away for a retreat. He needed to withdraw for a while, to stand back more objectively and examine his priorities again before God.

During their four days of silence, each person had the opportunity to speak for half an hour with the minister who had been leading their meditations.

"What would you like to talk about?" asked Peter, signaling Matthew toward a comfortable chair near the log fire.

"I need to howl at the heavens and hear you say 'There, there,'" replied Matthew. His voice was strangely bold in comparison with the rather desperate-sounding words he had chosen.

Peter did not stop to interrogate Matthew. "Howl away!" he suggested, but the furrow in his brow showed Matthew some of his bewilderment. Matthew was not put off. He was probably no less astonished himself at what he was saying. Rarely, if ever, had he shared so straightforwardly as he felt able to now.

"I've been the minister in my present congregation for eighteen months. It's a new church building in a new town: an ecumenical set-up with Christians of four different denominations all together. I find the whole situation very exciting. People who come to church say they like the style of worship. I feel I'm getting a handle on things. I have a vision of where I believe God wants to lead us, which is clear enough for me to have been able to set out distinct goals for the next five years."

Peter nodded, a quiet smile over his face as he shared Matthew's obvious happiness in what he was saying. A faint puzzlement remained, however, as he waited to hear more.

"I could talk of encouragement and tell you stories of different ways in which God has shown Himself in people's lives. But if I were to write out my work at the moment, I would need to slash a headline right across the page. It would read, 'THWARTED.' "

Peter's eyes did not leave Matthew's face.

"My wife, Jane, has a chronic debilitating illness. She has to bear a certain amount of pain every day. At times—perhaps twice a year—she develops new complications or new pockets of inflammation, each episode of which could become very serious or even fatal."

"How old is your wife?"

"She's thirty-one. She's had this—it's called pelvic inflammatory disease—for eleven years, ever since an appendix operation went wrong. She's had numerous operations for it, as you may imagine."

The compassion in Peter's eyes was such that he did not need to speak. "Whenever she's admitted to the hospital, as she was just recently, any timetable or plans for my own work are whisked away from me. The children need dressing, feeding, washing. I may snatch a couple of hours to myself here and there when Angus is at school and

Philippa's being looked after by some caring friend—but that's hopeless. The quality of those hours is dominated by other thoughts."

He looked up once again to Peter, whose expression was open and attentive. Matthew found his silence helpful, freeing him to speak without his words being criticized.

"Somehow I don't feel in charge anymore. I can no longer choose what I do—it's decided for me: organizing the children, shopping, cooking, answering the telephone . . . " He grunted and crossed his legs, jolting one leg strongly against the other as he began to recall so many interruptions to his work.

"What is the greatest tension?" asked Peter wisely, perceiving the spectrum of issues behind Matthew's words.

Matthew hardly needed to pause to answer. "I simply cannot reconcile the tension between the work which God has clearly called me to and the situation at home which equally clearly frustrates me from carrying out that work whenever Jane's unwell. You see, when I look at where God has put me, and I feel so pleased to be a round peg in a round hole, then everything seems so good and so right. I feel right where I am. But I feel torn in two. Twice since we came here eighteen months ago, Jane has had a fairly severe crisis which has put her out of action for weeks. Each time it has crashed right in on my work, inevitably cutting it down."

"How much help do you have for your home?"

"People in the parish are being particularly helpful at the moment. One person comes to the house for an hour or so each morning to do heavy work like cleaning, hanging out washing or whatever we ask. Another is taking Philippa regularly each week to give Jane an hour's guaranteed rest in the afternoon. Their help is marvelous; they've saved our bacon. But that sort of help is only temporarily bailing us out. Our situation is not temporary."

Matthew looked questioningly at Peter. Would a man such as he, a bachelor and wholly dedicated to his work as a minister, understand about the practical, mundane chores of deciding which clothes the children should wear or how frequently he had to remember Philippa's potty training?

Peter continued trying to grasp the whole of what Matthew wanted to howl at. "Can your relatives help?" he asked.

"My parents have dropped everything in order to come and stay with us for some weeks at a time. Since we've moved to Cheshire, Jane's mother lives nearer to us, and she could not have been more kind. Again, that has been marvelous in its own way while Jane's been at her lowest. But it does not stop me feeling torn and, well, invaded really."

Silence fell on the room. Matthew sat back in his chair, allowing the tension to ease a little now that he had put his feelings, which he still felt ashamed to speak out, into words. Was it selfish of him to be thinking of himself, when he was not the one to be bearing the physical pain? He closed his eyes, trying not to feel utterly condemned. He had seen no such condemnation in Peter's face as he had talked. It was his turn now simply to wait, listening attentively and prayerfully.

"It is no use waiting for a change in what is

happening *to* you. God wants you to offer what is happening *in* you," said Peter steadily.

Matthew did not hesitate in coming to the core of his frustration, "Can God be so tantalizing as to let me glimpse my vocation and then thwart me from fulfilling it?"

"God does not make unreasonable demands," Peter replied gently. "He asks you to give Him only what you can. At times, that may seem to us an offering far too small, sometimes second best. But God looks for us to offer our best in whatever work He has entrusted to us.

"Each of us is curtailed by certain limitations. One of your limitations is the health of your wife. But it is God who has given you first your wife, your family and then your work. It's quite fruitless for you to think, 'If only it weren't for Jane's illness I could do this, that and the other for God.' That is to expect yourself to give more to God than you are able to give."

Matthew was warmed by the unexpected reassurance of this man's words. He knew Peter was right. He had to embrace what had been inflicted upon him. He had to offer bathing the children as his service to God as much as visiting the sick in the congregation. The very thing he most wanted to offer to God he was to cast away.

It was quite contrary to his inclination, especially when some of his work looked so good, so full of promise. He had to trust God rather than hold on to what had seemed like God's work. He had to accept that even that wasn't for him to do now.

By the time he came home from his retreat, Matthew had resolved that he could offer his suffering as his ministry. He was infused with fresh peace. He knew that to suffer, on its own, was not a ministry. But to embrace the suffering which presented itself, and to give it to God, serving Him through it, was to embrace the fellowship of suffering for Christ. That was to fulfill his ministry.

Strangely, two of Matthew's church members — the very people whom Matthew would have wanted to "help" — were the ones who proved Peter's advice in practice. They demonstrated to Matthew and me how God transformed the most apparently insignificant things when they were offered to Him.

"Don't thank me," Maureen said almost every morning after I came home from the hospital as she put on her coat after spending an hour at the house doing the heavy housework.

"I can't *not* thank you, after all you've done," I replied equally regularly. I would point to the cleanly-swept floors, the washing hung out on the line to save my tummy stretching up, or the ironing neatly laid in piles.

"No, but I want you to understand, Jane," Maureen insisted last week. "It's not me you should be thanking, really. Honestly, it's God that does it. If He's given me a body that can do this, then there's nothing that will make me happier than to do it. I want to do what He wants me to do."

"But it helps me so very much. I feel that I would be ungracious if I didn't thank you. Even to thank you for doing what God wants," I insisted.

Maureen folded her arms and sighed. "Yes, I can see that. But I want you to know that I feel that you should be thanking God, not me. It's Him that's given me the body and the motivation to do it. If I take any thanks, I feel as if I'm stealing. Honestly, that's how strongly I feel." And her radiant eyes and glowing smile left no doubt in my mind that her humility was utterly genuine.

Lis is very similar. Twice every week she does our shopping in order to save me from yet another source of tiredness. For some months she also took Philippa to enable me not just to rest, but to sleep properly in bed. And she hates me to say I'm grateful to her.

"Don't say that," she chided kindly one day. "That sounds as if you feel indebted to me. It's not like that."

I may have taken after my mother in that I find it quite difficult to accept things from other people. We're both better at giving than receiving. So I heard myself reply, "But I do nothing in return for you!"

Lis, quiet by nature, sighed and leaned forward in her chair. She opened her mouth to speak, paused and then smiled a little. "You're just you," came her reply. I felt slightly embarrassed and unsure of how to reply, but decided to allow the silence to continue while she formulated the words to express what was on her mind.

At last she spoke again, "The other Sunday in church, we all had to ask ourselves what God wanted us to do to serve Him—remember?" I nodded. "Well, having just finished as church secretary, I had to think very hard what God wanted me to do. Did He really want me to do less, or just something different? I had to pray about it. But having done so, I now know that to help you in this way feels right. Even if it does sound odd to have a 'ministry of shopping,' or a 'ministry of child-minding'!"

She laughed and I joined in. What she had said rang true. I, too, had sometimes felt such a surge of God's peace as had Matthew. And because Lis offers to God her shopping for me, He has equipped her even to enjoy that ministry thoroughly. Like Maureen, she seeks no thanks and finds any gratitude I offer as an intrusion on her real reason for doing it, namely that it springs from her relationship with her Lord.

Matthew and I were learning the same lesson during my convalescence: The most useless things could become instruments in the hand of God. That was even apparent in someone so limited as to be paralyzed.

Since the age of seventeen, Joni Eareckson Tada has been paralyzed from the neck down. Matthew and I were enjoying the words of one of her songs as they drifted across the auditorium of Manchester's Free Trade Hall: "May I borrow your hands? They can work for me; together we'll do just fine . . . "

Joni raised her shoulders with all her effort, causing her splinted arms to be raised clumsily a few inches from the rests of her wheelchair. That was the only way she could cause her hands to move at all. She was almost entirely dependent on others' help.

I slid my gaze down to my own hands. One rested on Matthew's arm next to me; the other was clasped across my lower abdomen. That seemed to help the gnawing ache which was normal for me.

Only that afternoon I had longed to ask somebody the very same question. In order to use my hands I, too, had had to contort my body—but not because of paralysis. I had been trying to wash my hair in preparation to meet Joni. I was to present her with a copy of my book, and I wanted to look my best.

There was a cost. Raising the blow-drier to my dripping hair took a conscious effort. To lift my hands against the dragging ache was an act of will, quite contrary to my inclination. It stretched the scars from my operations. I grunted involuntarily as I finished, my arms flopping back down. For a few seconds I leaned my head on the dressing-table and waited for the worst waves of discomfort to subside.

"Not so very different from Joni," I had mused silently as I stared back to the mirror, hoping my efforts had been worthwhile. "Her hands are almost useless because of her paralysis. Mine are hampered by physical pain."

Those thoughts returned as I heard Joni's song. She was looking to her husband, Ken, as she asked for his help. He took her hand in both of his. But it was only because Joni was watching him that she could appreciate the squeeze he gave. For twenty years her hands had been able to feel nothing.

Just before the concert had begun, Matthew and I had been escorted backstage. There had been a bustle all around: Stewards checking the ramp for Joni's wheelchair; sound men rushing up to mend the amplification system. Radio reporters had stood with their microphones waiting to catch individual interviews with both Joni and myself. The atmosphere had been one of intense busyness.

We had been led from there into a poky little

dressing-room where, for a few minutes, we had been alone with Joni. We had shared how our pathways had been similar in many respects, though the circumstances different.

Before we had left her, Joni had taken a few minutes to savor the inscription I had written for her in the flyleaf of my book. During that pause I had become uncomfortable, knowing that our time together was strictly limited. Yet it had seemed inappropriate to rush our meeting. We had hardly needed words, but we did need time to appreciate the rapport between us.

Somebody had knocked on the door. The concert had already begun. Joni was due on stage. I had gotten up from my chair to leave.

But Joni would not be hurried. There was one question which she pressed me to answer.

"Jane, tell me," she had asked intently, as if oblivious to any pressure of time, "how do you cope with your pain, day by day?"

I had hesitated.

Why was Joni asking me that? Was she using a question to make conversation, trying to sound interested in me—a mark of her own gracious, generous personality? Had she not come to this concert to give us the answers? Or did she really want to know for herself?

I could have said quickly, "By praying, day by day." In one sense, that was true. But her honesty went deeper than such a quick generalization and I knew she would not have been satisfied. She would have wanted me to be more specific than that.

Perhaps I should have pointed her to the last

chapter of my book which rested on her knee now. That explained a little of Matthew's and my own everyday life. Yet I knew I had not managed to condense any one answer into that. We had already talked about my work on the sequel.

Through the glass panel of the door I could see pointed gesticulations toward the clock. I must not make Joni late. Yet her questioning eyes rested on me expectantly.

Pressured by time, I gestured to Matthew who had reached the door by now. The quiet support he gave was certainly one thing which helped me to cope. As we turned toward him, we both saw the urgent faces of those waiting outside and I knew Joni must get on stage.

Fumbling to give a quick reply, I could think of nothing but a straight answer. "I don't know," I spluttered. "I don't know!" Then, as the door had been opened for me, I had added more quietly, "But I guess it's more hour by hour than day by day."

Joni's eyes had twinkled as if she had understood, and I had hurried out. When I had peeped back through the door, her gaze had followed me and she had remained pensive and still, her head nodding assent.

"I hope you'll be better," she had called after me. I smiled back without conviction. I had been hoping that for the past eleven years. Seeing my expression, she bit her lip. She had not intended to sound glib.

She adjusted her words, "I mean, I hope at least it's better enough for you to concentrate on the rest of the program . . . " One of her helpers had released the brake of her wheelchair, and straight away she had had to turn her attention to getting on stage.

Now I pondered her question again as I listened to her tuneful singing. Clumsily she forced her splintered arm around a child. "May I borrow your hands?" she asked him cheerfully in song.

That was how she coped, day by day. Wherever she bumped into her limitations, she asked for a helping hand.

In that, I was different. I did not ask others to help me so freely as Joni. Sometimes, it was pride which held me back. I preferred to be seen as a coping person. I thought that asking for help was giving in. Only sissies gave in. I wanted to be brave and strong. At other times I was too afraid to ask, fearing that others might misuse the trust I put in them, and I shrank back from making myself vulnerable to their judgment. By doing so, I deprived those people of the opportunity to show their care. People like Jocelyn, whom I feared more than I trusted.

And of course, I had more freedom than Joni. I was not paralyzed. Yet I had to concede that I, too, needed help just to get me through some days.

I had never hesitated to ask God to help me. Undoubtedly He had provided answers to my pleas through others who acted as ambassadors for Him but, essential as they were in the throes of a crisis, that was not how I coped. They had helped on the outside, with the boring, necessary chores, but not deep within. Pain is one's own. Others can help, but it is only each individual who has, somehow, to bear it. It was the coping, hour by hour through the ongoing daily slog of pain with which I felt daunted.

I shuffled restlessly in my squeaky seat. How could I have answered Joni better, I wondered, when she had asked so sincerely how I coped?

I closed my eyes. How would my Lord have wanted me to answer? Tentatively, silently, I whispered to Him, "Lord, how do You want me to cope, day by day?" I determined to listen to Him.

Joni's tune played on. The words of the chorus were repeated once again and suddenly it was as if God Himself were posing the question through the words Joni was singing: "May I borrow your hands? They can work for me; together we'll do just fine."

It was not I who should be praying those words. It was my Lord! He is the One who lacks hands . . . hands to help, to reach out to others, to fulfill His work. He is the One who has no body on earth. Except, that is, for us. We are His body now.

With shame, I saw how I misuse Him when I ask Him to help me to achieve what I think is right. Whose work was I doing anyway? Or Matthew, in his pressure of ministry?

If we wanted to fulfill God's work, then we had no need to ask God to help us. It was God who longed for us to hear Him ask the very same question. Would we allow Him to use our hands? Our hands could work for Him. Our hands, however useless they seemed . . . There were Joni's hands, paralyzed and useless. But God was using them in their uselessness to fulfill His work in her. No matter how often my hands are clutched around my aching abdomen, it was as if He were asking if He might use them.

I looked around the auditorium. As it was for Joni, for myself, for Matthew, so, too, it was true for everyone else. It didn't matter how apparently use-less were so many pairs of hands as everyone sat there. Each pair of hands represented a different kind of pain: hands wrung together in anxiety; hands twisting wedding rings which had lost their meaning; hands stiff with old age; some hands covering tear-streamed faces. Were they, too, as-king God to help them?

However restricted we felt our hands to be, God had a use for them, even as they were. Day by day, hour by hour. To all of us, the miracle is that hearing Him thus is what helps us to cope.

Of course, Angus could have told me this from one of our precious conversations at his bedtime.

"God is here in this world, isn't He Mommy?" he had once asked.

"Yes, He is. He is everywhere."

"But He hasn't got a body?"

"No. When Jesus was alive He had a body. People could see Him. Jesus told them that everyone who had seen Him had seen God."

"*We* can't see Him now though, can we?"

"No. He's like the wind. How do you know when it's a windy day?"

"You can see!"

I shook my head. "It's so real, it may seem as if you can see it, but you can't, you know. Not the actual wind. You can see the trees bending, or your kite flying. But you can't see the wind."

"Mmm." He sounded unsure.

I puffed my breath gently on his face. "My breath is there, but you can't see it. You can feel it."

Angus giggled a little and reflattened his hair. "God is like that," I continued. "We can't see Him, but we know He's here. We have His power."

"I know we have His power," Angus became excited. I steeled myself, ready to hear God compared with Superman or some other television hero characterized by power.

But Angus surprised me: "God's power helps us to love."

I smiled. "Yes," I agreed, humbled that yet again a child should give such a mature perspective to a grown-up. "And He uses that power in us whenever we say we'll do what He wants. He hasn't got a body, but He uses ours."

8

Rocky Pathway

He makes my feet like the feet of a deer,
he enables me to go on the heights
(Habakkuk 3:19).

"Oh, Mrs. Grayshon, are you all right?"

The receptionist behind her desk at the health center was merely repeating a question asked by many others over the previous few weeks. So frequently since last being discharged from the hospital I had heard, "Jane, you look really tired." Matthew was even more direct: "You look grey."

But I had pushed away their caring comments. I felt I must force myself on, like a boat plowing a route through increasingly threatening ice to Antarctica, for which conditions become more and more difficult. The only hope, the only way through, I had thought, was to keep on moving. To wallow in my misery would do no good. Others would become bored if I always complained to them. I could not bear the loneliness of that.

During the few weeks since coming home from the hospital, I had expected to improve a little each day. Impatient to be better, I had gradually fulfilled more and more of my own responsibilities as wife and mother. Each day I had set myself new goals. I had done so very gradually, mostly because I knew my body was not ready to go at full speed. However, I was also aware that I had to be careful of what others would think.

Almost imperceptibly, I had increased my involvement. Matthew would still put laundry into the machine, but he would not necessarily notice that it had already been sorted into different loads. Maureen would still make the beds, but the bottom sheet would already have been smoothed or the nightclothes folded. Others would still bring food, but increasingly I was making my own side dishes. Such "independence" was important to my psychological well-being. The satisfaction and pleasure I derived benefitted me more than the drain on my physical resources. At least, so I believed.

Advice from all who constantly told me to "take it easy" washed straight over me. It sounded boring and I did not want to lead a boring life. It caused me to feel pressed into the mold of an invalid, and I did not want to be an invalid. I wanted to resist that. I chose to ignore their advice. I struggled on.

Thus it was no surprise to me to hear the receptionist at the health center ask, "Are you all right?" It had become routine for me to reply that I was.

I had spoken to the doctor on the telephone

earlier, but had been unable to find the right words to describe adequately how I felt. In any case, I had become increasingly afraid of boring him, moaning drearily on each time I saw him. It had been a mark of his understanding that he had asked me to let him assess how I was for himself. And so I had slipped down to the health center.

It was not until I stood facing the receptionist that the cold in my hands spread with a rush over my whole body. I tried to grip on to her desk as her face seemed to disappear into an ever-shrinking hole before my eyes. The world turned grotesquely black.

Suddenly I was aware of people all around me, above me. I desperately wanted to get a breath, but something was blocked. I could not move. They seemed to be pushing me, handling my body. I was utterly limp. Once again—yet again—I had been catapulted into the position I loathed.

"On her side," instructed the doctor, slightly breathless after being summoned hastily from his room. I was pushed over. At last that movement jerked my tongue forward. With relief I gasped a breath. Still the world was black.

"Her pulse is picking up now." The doctor's voice sounded steadied. He was able to reassure himself, if not the onlookers.

Slowly, gradually, their voices became less echoing. At last I found myself able to move one leg. It seemed an obvious priority to get myself out of the exposed position in which I was lying. I pushed my dress down.

Still they talked about me and I was unable to

join in. They decided to take me to a more appropriate room. Someone tried to lift me.

"No!" I found my voice to interject. I had never allowed myself to be carried, not even on one occasion when I had been so seriously ill I had been on the brink of dying. "I'll walk."

Those were the only words I spoke. Everything else seemed to wash over me, quenched by the waves of pain and discomfort in my abdomen. I had been lying on a couch for some minutes when the doctor was above me again, fumbling for a word.

"Oh yes. I've got it," he said, looking satisfied. "Dictatorial."

"What?" I asked, still stupefied. What was he talking about?

"Dictatorial," he repeated. "That's what I'm going to be." I looked away from him. I must have sensed what he was about to say and I did not want to face it. But that did not prevent him from continuing. "I want you to be seen by the specialist while you are as you are now. You're going to the hospital."

I turned my back to him and opened my mouth to argue, but he raised both hands to stop me. He spoke first. "Now, there's no arguing, no discussion, no buts. I've decided and that's it."

I saw that this was no time for me to dispute with him. A fighter by nature, I had resisted being admitted to the hospital for weeks previously, and he himself had most generously supported me in that question, for much longer than he may have liked. But now I had been stripped of the ability to fight back. Once again I saw no way of escape other than to follow down the old path I loathed so much.

I had to hold back the tears of distress and frustration which longed to be shed.

The doctor must have understood the wretchedness I felt, for he dropped the very firm note to his voice which he had had to assume in order to assert his authority. "I'm sorry," he said kindly. "You know yourself, really though, don't you? You just don't like to admit it." He smiled compassionately. "Brain over body, that's what you want. Well your body has won today." He paused. "I mean, you didn't tell me you felt this bad when you spoke to me earlier, did you?"

I did not answer. Poor man. He had an uphill task with me as one of his patients. I did not always understand myself why I was like that. Anyway I did not need to reply.

"End of a good friendship," he said as he left, but the amicable squeeze to my arm told me he didn't mean it.

But my mind was neither distracted nor consoled, not even by his caring manner. I was so consumed with revulsion for the hateful position in which I found myself that I could think of nothing else. Only once did I open my eyes, when my face was hit by the crisp air outside as I was wheeled into the ambulance. Branches of silver birch tree were silhouetted sharply by the clear blue sky. Then the world of normality was shut out again as the doors were slammed shut. We sped down the streets and I could only see the world through the darkened windows. I was encased in a different world: the private world of pain.

Once again I had to accept the horribly predictable pattern of my illness. I would just get over one bout and begin to get into the swing of life. I would take the risk of making new commitments, start becoming more involved again at church and do more of the extra, optional activities with our children when, *woomph,* I would go down again. More illness, more hospitalization, more pain. It was as if a machine had been programmed whose course had to be followed: hospital admission, questioning, X-rays, more questioning.

Incessantly I was questioned. What had happened today? During the past few weeks? How had all this started? What exactly had been done at each of the operations I had had? First the nurses, then the technicians and the staff in the X-ray department all had their repertoire with their statutory forms to fill out. Why did they have to keep asking me? Couldn't they read the catalogue of operations in my notes? It was not so long since my previous admission. I resented the intrusion that their interrogation caused. I felt fragile enough already without such an onslaught.

The specialist was in his outpatient clinic and it was decided that I could be examined by him there. I may not have to be admitted. In his letter my GP had simply asked for him to assess me. I waited apprehensively for him to come in.

I thought back to the night in that same hospital when the decision had been to watch and wait. I had missed an operation by a hair's breadth. The surgeon, convinced I had another pelvic abscess, had been all ready to open me up in the middle of the night.

I was very fortunate. Our GP knew of the need to hold back on surgery for as long as possible. He and the specialist, Geoff, had both taken a personal interest in my case. Not only had they taken the time to read the lengthy details of my history when we had first moved to their area, but they worked together. They even prayed together about me! And so it had been, in the middle of that night, that as soon as the ambulance had whisked me off to the hospital, the GP had made personal contact with Geoff at his own home.

This time it was my turn to be perturbed. I felt worse now than I had then. I determined not to conceal any symptoms today, whatever the consequences.

"How are you doing?" Geoff's voice echoed hollowly around the white-walled room. He was still writing notes from the previous patient. I had a few seconds to think how to reply.

At last he was ready to hear. "How are you doing?" he repeated his enquiry when he had completed his flurrying signature.

I smiled, uncomfortable at being faced so straight with the question I loathe so much to answer. "I'm not sure," I replied hesitantly. "I suppose I don't think I'm very well, actually."

"Come on." He walked swiftly to the other end of the examination room. "Let me have a look at you." He patted the examining table and began to draw the curtains around it. Then, when I struggled to my feet, he added, "Take your time."

Soon we were back in our places, he at his desk and me on the chair beside him. He began to record his findings in my notes and complete the various forms for blood tests.

"Any questions?" he asked kindly, but without looking up.

There were so many questions in my mind that I found it hard to put them into words, especially because I had to be swift. The line of other patients outside the door was acting as a pressure on our conversation. We both knew his clinic was running very late.

I leaned forward uncomfortably on my chair. Geoff seemed, from his manner, to take things so much in his stride that I was afraid I had maybe not been candid enough in telling him how unwell I felt. He had not commented on his observations and I did not want to leave him with a false impression of fitness.

I tried to articulate my question objectively. "I must say, I think there's something wrong . . . " I began. It was new for me to hear myself put my complaints so directly.

Geoff looked up and frowned, as if I had misunderstood his invitation. "We know there's something wrong," he stated, smiling slightly at my naivete.

"What I'm saying is, I feel . . . " I cleared my dry throat, "I feel as if there's something there . . . "

His puzzled frown remained and he said quickly, "We know there's something there. There is infection there. Your peritoneum is inflamed again." He spoke without emotion, though he was as friendly as always. Then he resumed his writing.

I was slightly stunned. Such a diagnosis wasn't good. Why did he not seem at all perturbed? His voice was so calm. Perhaps it was that casualness which I found most difficult. Or was he falling into my own trap of concealing any reaction he may have had behind a smile?

After a pause I spoke again. At least I felt at ease to share with him what was troubling me.

"You remember you've said before that you'd be hesitant to do a laparoscopy . . . ?" This specially small instrument would allow him to see what was going on inside my abdomen with only a minor incision.

Before I had even finished my sentence, Geoff's hand froze where he had been writing. He flinched and shut his eyes, as if blocking off the very possibility, the mere thought, of such an absurd idea.

I pressed him further. "Well, what would it take—I mean, how bad do I have to be before you do decide to have a look?" I pursued. I could not be confident that everything was under control unless Geoff had seen exactly what was going on.

"I don't need to have a look," he responded. "I'm sure I'd find pus in there." His manner was less hasty now. Perhaps he could see that I was having difficulty in realizing how much he understood, but was unable to cure.

He completed the forms in silence. I felt numb. I was unable yet to take in what he was saying, never mind respond. It seemed scarcely credible to me that I could have such a severe infection; especially because, from the smile on Geoff's face, I would never have known . . .

For a second when Geoff looked up from his writing, I saw a tiny image of myself reflected in his spectacles.

"Well," he explained gently, helping me to see

his rationale. "That's what has been found before, and there's every indication that it's there again today. But the point about a laparoscopy is that, even when that's been done in the past and pus had been identified, nobody has ever been able to do anything about it in surgery. There's no point in putting you through the risk of even further trauma just for me to see it with my own eyes." For the first time he frowned, hesitating. "A laparoscopy could do untold damage. Do you realize that?"

In my helplessness, I answered flippantly, "You could pray." But such a comment reflected more my own impotence and fear than any spirituality.

"I'm quite sure now of what I would see," he replied. "An inflamed abdomen and peritoneum, pockets of pus, adhesions . . . "

I sat motionless and thoughtful. He turned to write a prescription. "I'm giving you two different antibiotics for at least six months," he said, explaining about each one as he wrote, "and I want you to take these others as well." He scribbled his signature and, tearing the page off the pad, passed all the forms across to me. "A minimum of six months," he emphasized. I nodded.

"I don't need to have you admitted if you behave yourself at home. You'd be better off feeling as you are at home than in here. I'll hear how you're getting on via the GP."

My thanks for that were sincere.

"And my nausea?" Feeling sick made me feel thoroughly dragged down.

He put his fingertips together and leaned his chin on his two forefingers. "That's not the main problem," he said. "Just a complication. There's no obstruction at the moment, but what's probably happening is that, around the actual site of the inflammation and pus, you're forming a small ileus—a loop of bowel which is temporarily paralyzed and seized up."

It sounded as uncomfortable as I felt. "So that's what is causing me to feel sick?" I asked.

"Yes."

"And you're not bothered about that?"

He hesitated before answering, flicking his front teeth with his thumb. "You're not actually vomiting, are you?"

"No."

"Then that's all right. No, I'm not worried about the nausea."

"Rotten doctors!" I muttered. He giggled. "I complain of a horrible, debilitating symptom and you're not bothered unless I produce vomit!"

Both of us were laughing now, but a part of me was uncomfortable within our mirth. It was confusing. Was it inappropriate? Perhaps our surface merriment was the only way we could both cope.

A nurse brought Geoff a cup of coffee, whispering that Matthew had arrived and if I was not to be staying in the hospital, he would be able to take me home.

From what she saw of our merriment, that nurse could have had no idea of what was going on. It must have been incongruous to her that Geoff had just diagnosed peritonitis in me. She never would have known.

"Keep in touch with me," Geoff told me as I

made my way to the door. "I need to know if you do start vomiting because it's a sign of true obstruction. If that does happen, then of course I shall have to free those adhesions causing it."

Inwardly, I sighed, feeling increasingly trapped. Outwardly, I reciprocated Geoff's smile and left the room.

That evening, once the children were peacefully settled in bed, I slipped downstairs to my little praying corner, even though my body ached with tiredness. I wanted to try to drink in some of God's peace.

As a gesture of my sincerity in wanting to draw near to God, I lit a candle on a low shelf. I shook out the match's flame and glanced at the notes huddling in a pile near the candle. There were many cards or precious letters—ones which I had kept and treasured because they helped me to focus my prayers. Philippa's special "bread" stone from Arisaig had taken its place there, too.

Perched against the wall at the back was one such letter written on a pale blue card. At the top I had glued a picture of flagstones making a pathway across a field brightly adorned with poppies; the other half of the page bore writing. One dear and trusted friend—a lady much older than myself, and with wisdom and maturity I admired—had been moved to write after spending some time praying specifically for Matthew and myself. She had passed them on with a loving note to us, believing them to be inspired directly by the Holy Spirit. She had written more than a year ago, but I had kept her letter to dwell on at my leisure.

I picked up the page and read the words once again:

> My children,
> You are Mine.
> You are not alone.
> Neither are you free to go your own way.
>
> You are Mine.
> My love is over you.
> I will never leave you.
> In submission to Me you will find
>   freedom and joy.
> You are Mine.
>
> Walk in My path, My children.
> I will light your way.
>
> Do not be distracted by flowers in the fields.
> Keep going steadily along My path.
> On My path you will find rest and joy . . .

There I tripped over the words and stopped. My eyes rested longingly on the word *joy*.

If this friend had truly been prompted by the Holy Spirit, then God was telling me that I would find joy. And the promise was for the joy, not by being released from the pain of my pathway, but right on it: "On My path you will find rest and joy."

There was such promise and confidence, all my hopes and aspirations were caught up in the words. But "His path"? Could I be sure that the pain I had to face was part of His path?

I looked back over the page, searching to understand. Joy seemed such an inappropriate word to describe what lay along a painful path. Surely there was no joy in accepting stones like the one which now glinted in the soft candlelight? Yet as I scanned the poem, my eye fell on it again, higher up the page. "In submission to Me you will find freedom and joy . . . "

But how could I submit to Him when He persistently withheld healing? How could that be freedom, when it wounded only like a trap? Oh, I knew God had reassured me frequently that He was with me through whatever pain I had to face. But that was different from asking me to *submit* to the idea of such pain. The very thought of that kind of submission made me feel like a slave. To do so seemed to ask me to lie down to be trampled on. Where was the freedom in that? And joy?

"Lord, what is this?" I begged Him suddenly to answer me. The blue piece of card in front of me was no longer just poppies decorating a printed page. The words began to be God speaking, and I felt I could reply to Him. I covered my eyes and buried my face in my hands.

It felt so unjust. "Listen, Lord," I bargained, as if He did not already know what I was about to say, "I believe You when You speak. I trust You. And I have tried hard to keep trusting that You haven't made some mistake, that You haven't overlooked the fact that pain is such a prominent part of my life. Many others think I'm crazy to keep trusting You. How can You possibly talk about me finding 'rest and joy' or 'freedom and joy' when things are so grim?"

I bent forward as I knelt, until my face was near to the floor. It was not just with tears that I was bowed down. Somewhere deep within, I wanted to prostrate myself before my Lord—even physically— and listen to His answer. I was glad to be alone in the house, so I could be unafraid of being caught in a foolish-looking posture. I needed to bare my soul to Him, to be honest toward Him, and for that I needed to be uninhibited and alone.

The gentle fragrance of the candle in front of me filled the air even as I breathed. I opened my eyes, kneeling up straighter to settle my eyes on it. The flame did not flicker. It remained unfaltering and steady.

My mind became calmer and my questionings hushed. I could sense the steady, unfaltering character of God. I closed my eyes once more and opened my hands toward Him. Softly, quietly, I found myself weeping gentle tears.

More quietly now, I prayed, "Show me Your rest, Lord. If I can't have rest from the pain, show me rest within it. Not somewhere else, but right where I am. On my pathway, my rocky pathway, show me Your joy."

My tears may have been similar to those of Sarah in her mourning. Similar, no doubt, to Jocelyn's, to Mary's, maybe to everybody's in the secrecy of their own hearts. But it was Sarah's faltering voice I could hear repeating in the recesses of my mind, "Do you believe in the goodness of God?"

Then, hesitantly, as if to explain to my own Father, I garbled, "This pain isn't what I want. It doesn't seem like Your goodness. But yes, I do believe in Your goodness. Forgive me for thinking You would offer a stone instead of bread."

The circle of wax around the wick grew bigger and, as it did so, tiny black flecks separated out, drawn toward the flame as if by a magnet.

"If You're not going to take the pain away from me, please help me to accept it. Help me to reach out and receive whatever You give. Help me to see whatever You give as bread and not stones. Help me to feed on You, Lord. And show me Your freedom, even if pain goes on and on . . . "

For some moments I remained, kneeling before the Lord. The candle's vapors wafted upwards in silence.

I sighed resignedly as I got up at last. Admittedly I did feel more peaceful having spent time in prayer, but I had found no resolution which satisfied me. My wrestling remained. I would have to wait to discover God's secrets as the days unfolded.

9

Whose Harvest?

*Those who wept as they went out carrying
the seed will come back singing for joy, as
they bring in the harvest (Psalm 126:6, GNB).*

A letter lay on the table awaiting my return
from taking Angus to school. It was one of many
each week which I had come to welcome from those
who had either heard me on the radio or who had
read my story. Sometimes our friends wrote encouragingly. More often I heard from people whom
I had never met.

Matthew, at the opposite side of the table, was
slitting open his own pile of letters in a leisurely
manner. Still tired from biking, I perched one leg on
a kitchen stool for a moment, undoing the zipper of
my jacket. I would just skim the short letter hastily
to glean the gist of it, before getting on with the
morning's jobs.

I glowed with pleasure as I read. The note was

119

a simple one of thanks, telling me how much my talk had meant when I had come to this lady's church. I felt encouraged by her sincerity and looked forward to relishing her words properly at a more convenient moment.

Then I turned over the page and found myself paying more thoughtful attention.

> I also want to tell you that, from where I was looking on Sunday, indeed "not one hair on your head has been singed." You shone with radiance from the Lord as you spoke to us, and no one could be in doubt about that extra person in the "furnace" with you.

I gazed pensively at the simple handwriting. With a final loving "thank you," the writer had signed off. That was all she had said.

Matthew looked up from his second cup of coffee. "Good mail?" he asked casually.

Smiling quietly, I passed him the letter. I wanted to share any pat on the back which came my way. He was so bound up with me in the day-to-day slog of my pain and limitations, he needed every bit of encouragement as I did that God's hand was on us even through the pain.

He gave my hand an affectionate squeeze as he read. "That's lovely," he said warmly, passing back the page. "Straightforward, sincere encouragement. Just lovely."

He was right. The encouragement was lovely. He dashed off to his study. And I felt terribly alone. For a moment, I gave no thought to pursuing the suspicious silence of Philippa upstairs—whatever mischief she might have found. I picked up the second page again. I stared at its neat writing. Why could I not see it to be true?

I settled myself more comfortably at the break-fast bar and pictured the quaint, squat church and the large, welcoming fellowship Matthew and I had visited a couple of weeks earlier. A slightly plump lady with a jolly, smiling face had read the Old Testament story from Daniel about the fiery furnace.

I had chosen the reading because my own experience was similar to that of Shadrach, Meshach and Abednego. The "fire" in which I found myself was not literally a furnace, but at times the pain had taken on an intensity which could only be described as being like a fire.

Like Shadrach, I was certain that God could have saved me from the furnace, had He chosen to do so. With Shadrach, I could have said, "The God we serve is able to save us" (Daniel 3:17). But in that Old Testament story, God had not chosen to deliver those men from the furnace. And He had not saved me from my illness. The miracle had been different. Despite the intense heat of the furnace, they had not been consumed by the fire.

Wanting to listen attentively to the particular part of the reading which I found so inspiring, I stopped following the passage in my own Bible. I watched the lady in her blue dress lean her arms on the huge church Bible. With awe I heard her read that when Nebuchadnezzar had looked, he had seen not just three, but four men. The fourth had looked like the Son of God.

I had raised my head to ponder the words. How I wanted God to be seen in me, too! Silently I began to pray that He would be—even that morning, even though I still felt in a "furnace" of long-term pain—

and I asked God that those people listening would see Him, too.

The lady in her blue dress had not quite reached the end. In those last moments before it was my turn to speak, I was suddenly jolted out of my quiet thoughts. With glorious conviction she read, "The fire had not harmed their bodies, nor was a hair of their heads singed; their robes were not scorched, and there was no smell of fire on them" (Daniel 3:27).

My heart sank. When preparing my talk beforehand, I had not especially noticed that sentence. And that meant that the similarity ceased between my experience and theirs. It was not true for me that the fire had not harmed my body. How could I now speak of my own experience as being parallel? I wanted to be honest and truthful.

But I had no time to think, for within a few moments I was standing in the pulpit and sharing the story of my own pilgrimage through a fiery furnace.

"I know that, as God was with Shadrach, Meshach and Abednego in the furnace, so He has been with me," I said. "He did not preserve them from the fire, and He has not saved me from peritonitis." I told them how I had nearly died. Some sat back into their pews, blinking back tears they were too deeply involved to conceal.

"His miracle in me has been to rescue me not *from* it but *within* it—by being with me, in it—as He was with Shadrach and his friends." I told them of my experience in Beverley.

"I know that others are more able to see Him with me and with Matthew, than we can ourselves."

My voice became quiet now, and nobody stirred. And then, before I was able to stop myself, I found myself admitting to everybody, "But the ending of our story is different." My voice faltered. "I wish I could share the same happy ending, but if I'm honest, I can't say that God has protected us from being singed or from having any smell of fire upon us."

Matthew's distinctive suit jacket near the front of the church drew my gaze over to him. His arms were folded and he was listening as attentively as everyone else.

"Sometimes, I look at Matthew and at how he is affected when I am in a lot of pain. That is very hard. I feel as if he is the one who smells the fire as he takes the consequences of my hard times . . . "

Now, reading that letter, I frowned. Leaning my elbows on the table I turned it over repeatedly in my hand, willing that second page to be true. "From where I was looking on Sunday, indeed 'Not one hair on your head has been singed.' You shone with radiance from the Lord as you spoke to us . . . "

Was it possible that I could shine? Really shine? I gave a heavy sigh. I wanted to believe so. I had prayed for God's glory to be seen, if not by a healing miracle, then in the midst of it all.

But something in me hung back from trusting there to be a purpose to such awful pain. However kindly she had surely meant it, hadn't this correspondent put me on to a glorious pedestal? Indulging in sentimentality, whitewashing suffering into something pleasantly victorious?

And worst of all, a new doubt crept into my thinking. Was I doing the same? Was writing a book just some pathetic way of making something as futile as chronic pain seem worthwhile? The question horrified me. I despised the idea that I could have sunk to such desperate, deluded rationale.

At first it was just a niggle: "You can't believe that pain is as fruitful as this morning's letter suggested . . . " Gradually, however, it grew inside until soon it became a voice which taunted me: "You know underneath how futile pain is, so what's the point in writing? A harvest from pain indeed!"

I did not recognize whose was the voice who would taunt me like that. The question was so cunningly put that it felt true. Increasingly, I felt accused. I had been gullible and naive. The words which had been so sincerely written to encourage me began instead to haunt me.

Yet somewhere in the recesses of my mind, her words found an echo. At some other time I had read this sort of message. That evening I searched along my bookshelf and picked out a file.

I flipped through it and pulled out an old letter. It had been written by a friend, John, back in 1980 when I had been critically ill. But his words held my attention as much now as they had then: "I touch Christ when I see you. I touch Him when I see the marks of Christ's suffering and victory in you," he had written. "You are the aroma of the very presence of Christ . . . "

How could John write that? For I am not the holy person his words suggested. Wasn't his use of the words rather extravagant? A measure of his Christ-like nature, always finding the best in others? I allowed myself to savor his encouraging sentiment for a few indulgent moments before sifting through more notes.

Soon my flipping across the corners of the pages stopped. Yes, there among the various book reviews was the comment which I was searching for: "Nobody reading this book or hearing Jane address a meeting in the visible frailty of her body could mistake Who is at the center of her life, Whose she is, or where she is going. It is about a life illuminated by Christ . . . Thank you, Jane."

Illuminated . . . shining. They were lovely words, and both reflected the description of Shadrach and his friends shining to God's glory in their furnace. But they were written by people who had seen only one side of me. Even if they could have been true, they were not the whole truth. There was another side, too, which was exactly the opposite.

For the following few days the mocking, cynical voice inside me seemed to take every opportunity to point out my every blemish. One incident in particular served to confirm the condemnation of myself. At our own church I felt cut right down by a lady who had an enormous amount of pain in her life—pain very different from mine, but no less real and probably much more intense. She was bitterly aware of the grind of suffering, on and on. Almost every relationship in her life was a difficult and uphill struggle for her to endure. Matthew often referred to her as "a walking miracle" because she had survived through so much.

When I had greeted her cheerfully, she refused to reciprocate my smile. She must have felt slapped in the face by me. *It's all right for her,* she seemed to be thinking. *Going off speaking about suffering or doing her glamorous television and radio programs.* Her eyes narrowed and she turned away. Just the sight of me was provocative.

I felt stunned. Her back was like a reproach to me. "You see now, Jane?" that inner voice lost no time in jumping in. "If you were authentic and there were really a harvest, then that woman would be thanking you for helping her to see God in her furnace. And is she? Ha ha!" it mocked. "Just look at her back turned against you!"

I became more and more ground down. The letter earlier in the week seemed a world away, its praise quite inappropriate to one so rotten as myself. "You shone with a radiance from the Lord." She would not have said that had she seen me now, I thought.

Once or twice I broached the subject with friends and oh, they said nice things to counter-balance my gloom. But the cynical voice allowed me no consolation. After all, they were friends. Friends are supposed to be fans.

For about a week I turned the letter over in my mind. By then I wanted to ignore the questions it raised in me. I was trying to write this book, and I was plagued with the idea that my writing was merely a pitiful attempt to drag some worth out of my suffering.

Then one morning, determined to get the manuscript completed, I sat down at my desk as usual to try to write. Once more, the right words would not come. I could not focus my mind properly on what I wanted to say. It was as if any creativity had been blocked, choked out by other distracting, self-centered thoughts. I felt sick—not just physically but mentally, too.

I put down my pen and gazed at the papers all over my desk. Writing was a lonesome job; it had to be. The children had both been taken to the zoo, and Matthew was out visiting. While usually I welcomed such peace to work, that morning my aloneness became strangely lonely.

A telephone call from a friend, Gill, was a welcome interruption. To hear her was a relief. I had wanted someone to turn to and say how I felt. I told her of my confusion.

"Of course, it's Satan who makes false accusations," she said quickly. She sounded rather witheringly casual and matter-of-fact. "He wants you to get fed up about your pain because it's his business to stop us from seeing God's loving hand in our lives. He wants all of us to feel that everything's futile, and most especially those things which would bring glory to God. It's his subtle way of making us feel fed up with God."

I had not thought of this. My inability to see any fruit had all seemed so justified, so reasonable, I had not considered that the old devil would poke his big nose in and distort my thinking.

"But hang on," I reasoned. "How do you know it's him? What I'm saying might be true!"

"Well, it sounds to me as if there's a lot of self-doubt and false accusation going around. That's a clear mark of Satan's big boots interfering."

"Oh, honestly!" I exclaimed wearily. I felt rather daunted at the prospect of facing battles on yet another front. "So what am I supposed to do with all these arguments floating around my head?"

"Well," Gill sounded as if she was stating the obvious, "whenever you feel taunted you say to yourself, 'God is with me.' And you can think of specific verses from the Bible, or any other signs He may have given you that He is with you. Then you just tell the devil to go away and leave you alone!"

I envied Gill's refusal to be intimidated by the devil and her ability to keep him so firmly in his place—at least, in this instance.

"Yes," I conceded. "But what about my writing? What if that's some pathetic attempt to bring supposedly 'good' things, like a book, out of what is actually miserable, futile pain? Perhaps I should listen to those doubts and chuck it all."

"Which is exactly what Satan wants," Gill completed my logic for me. "You know perfectly well that your 'doubts' are not true. Satan is a liar. He'd do anything to stop glory being given to God, whether it's through your writing or whatever anyone offers for God."

Gill was right. God accepts whatever I give to Him. It's Satan who tries to make my offerings seem worthless, not good enough. "God can never use that!" he scoffs.

I put the phone down and gazed out to the garden just in front of my window. I had been so busy looking for God's help that I had been lulled away from that precious closeness with my Lord. I had been deceived into thinking that, if there were any harvest from my pain such as that lady had written about, it was my own. A part of me had accepted credit which had really belonged to God.

I closed my eyes. "I'm sorry, Lord," I prayed quietly. "I undermine what You do. You know how rotten I am inside . . . " I looked up again at the crocuses pushing their way up through the soil.

"Be bigger in me, Lord. Make me willing for You to be seen more, for me to point to You rather than to me. I do not shine. I am rotten inside. Yet You shine in me. Thank You that You do bring good things even from what seems so worthless, that You do bring glory to Yourself even if I try to steal that very glory from You."

I gave a sigh and dragged my thoughts back to the work in front of me. Could I dare to go on writing?

From the buff-colored folder, the dark felt-tip lettering of the title stared up at me: *A Harvest From Pain.* Yes, I conceded. A harvest is not something unusual or spectacular. We are not surprised when seeds grow into mature plants. That's just normal — the natural consequence of sowing seeds.

It is the same with the seeds which are sown within my pain — everybody's pain. If there is any fruit, that is nothing unusual. It is not an achievement for which I should be praised. It is merely a product of growth — my life in God. As with any harvest, the extent to which a plant grows and bears fruit depends on the life-giving sap which rises from the depths, plumbed by its roots.

The trauma of the previous week gradually settled into its right perspective. What had felt vulnerable and raw became a fresh openness to God. With relief I could accept that I am no different from everyone else in their pain. God is seen in all those who offer their suffering to Him. All He asks is for me to look to Him within the pain. He does all the rest. He causes the fruit to grow. I just watch in amazement and thankfulness whenever I glimpse that fruit.

"The answer to your question to Matthew was

right in front of us!" A businessman was shaking my hand warmly after Matthew and I had preached together on Sunday.

I looked at him quizzically, a little unsure of what he meant. He was smiling warmly as he continued, "You said that God is able to do far more abundantly than ever we ask or think, and you asked Matthew for an example. Well," and he cupped both hands around mine, "we just had to look at you to see the example. You are the living example. We could see His Spirit pouring out from you. That is so special. It's 'far more abundant' than any physical healing that you may have asked Him for!"

I thanked that man for his encouragement, not knowing how often I would think back to it.

Is it pride for me to believe him? Only if I take it as a compliment to myself—which it was not. He was not referring to my courage, my strength, my supposed bravery in the face of my struggle. He was man enough to know that I frequently feel far from brave.

No. The compliment was to my Lord, to the One who chooses to live and work in me, even me. Even when I do not ask Him, He generously gives to me, blessing me in areas of my life which I may not even recognize. Even when I fail to thank Him—just like nine of the ten lepers—He graciously heals me. He does so because that is His nature. His goodness is imponderable.

The privilege for me is that I have actually been told what everyone deserves to know . . . That even if God is not removing their pain, He is doing "far more abundantly" than ever they could ask or even think of.

The privilege for me is of being given a glimpse into others' suffering—suffering which is normally kept carefully hidden away. But it is there. Everyone, in his turn, has his own kind of pain. Everyone has some idea of what it is like to be cast into a burning, fiery furnace. And when we dare face that, and accept it, we can see that we are not alone. We become aware of others in their furnace of different pain. And when we allow God in with us, then we can be given the very encouragement for which we crave: that God is glorified because He is visible in us.

10

Temptation (II): Hard Hearts

The Lord saw, and grieved . . . and His heart was filled with pain (Genesis 6:6).

Pain may be all-consuming to ourselves. Others, seeing only the harvest it yields, may only glimpse it.

No one ever could have guessed that Clara knew pain so deeply. Perhaps we should have recognized that she was able to understand and draw alongside the patients in a special way. Had I had more maturity in my days as a student nurse, I might have recognized that the quality of compassion which was natural to her had grown with much struggle from seeds of pain.

Clara had been fun to work with on the wards, and she was a bright student. Throughout our years of training together, she did outstandingly well. But she never accepted praise. Although nominated as

"Nurse of the Year," she declined to stand for election.

"That's not what nursing's about!" she chided an old lady affectionately one day. I glanced up at her across the ward from where I was taking temperatures. Clara did not know I had overheard and was watching her so carefully. Her eyes twinkled as she tucked a pillow comfortably underneath an old lady's swollen leg. No. She was content to know that she cared as she felt best. She nursed conscientiously because that was what she loved, and such dedication showed.

After we had all graduated—and Clara's diploma was etched in red to pronounce her distinction—her good reputation spread. The patients warmed to her, confided in her, loved her. Within a few years she flew to a developing country where she used her skills more widely.

Years later Clara came to stay with us on one of her visits back to Britain. Among the treasures she was showing me, she came across a note tucked inside a beautiful, hand-carved wooden box.

Thin lines of black ink scrawled across the back of the postcard. "May I read it?" I asked, intrigued by the unsteady hand.

Clara beamed. "Of course," she agreed. Her face lit up. "It's from one of my patients—an old man who had come in from the country. The hospital was all very strange to him. But I think I helped . . . "

She paused to allow me to read: "This carving is a token of my thanks to you, Sister. You have had a profound effect on me. You are one of those people one could never forget. I am grateful to God for the faith which He has increased in me through you. Thank you."

I handled the postcard carefully. I felt humbled and unsure of what to say to Clara. I wanted to endorse what that man had said, but my words would only have sounded clumsy alongside his.

"Clara, what a wonderful tribute!" I looked over to her sitting cross-legged on the floor. She had not yet accustomed herself to chairs again after her years on simple mats.

Clara smiled rather distantly.

"Don't you think so?" I pressed for her to join in my enthusiasm. "I mean, that's a lovely thing to have said about you! It must be one of the most heartwarming letters you've ever received."

Clara nodded vaguely. Something in her expression unsettled me. She slipped the postcard back silently into the box with which it had come.

I frowned, impatient for her to speak.

"Goodness, I'd be over the moon if I had a letter like that. I'd get Matthew to frame it for me!"

She snapped the lid closed.

"What's wrong?" I pressed. I could not understand why she was not as thrilled as I was. She was usually very bubbly in her enthusiasm. "Why are you hiding it? Anyone would think you were ashamed of it . . . "

At last she looked up. Her face was scored with anxiety.

"I think I am," she said slowly.

I was silenced. The pop-popping of the gas fire

beside us suddenly sounded very noisy. Clara un-
crossed her legs, hugging them instead to her chest.

"I'm not that special," she said. "If he admires
me so much I must have done something wrong—
manipulated him in some way. I can't trust that sort
of thing. Unless of course he wants something."

I was astonished. I had never doubted Clara's
self-confidence. I had always thought she knew her
strengths so well. She seemed able to accept them
and build on them. Why did she doubt her worth
when she was so complimented?

I thought back to the days when we had worked
together, to that occasion when she had refused to
be Nurse of the Year. Something in her manner had
unsettled me then. It was not just that she had been
self-effacing. There had been a trace of tension, of
fear. It had been as if she were afraid that such
praise was all a mean joke which could only hurt
her.

I had raised the subject later that day when we
were dragging off our starched uniform aprons.
Clara was struggling to undo the stud fastening her
collar and her chin was raised to allow room for her
fingers to fiddle at it. Wretched things! They almost
choked us. But I sensed that that had not been the
only reason for her voice to sound so strained.

"No—please don't!" And I felt bound to respect
the signals she gave that the matter was closed. I
concluded that this was one more sign of her lovely
nature: a rightful guard against pride.

But her reaction now, though it was years later,
disquieted me still. Was she unable to trust praise?
Did she always have to reject it?

"Clara, that note is straightforwardly appreciative. Why can't you just enjoy his admiration of you?"

She shook her head. Tears filled her eyes and I knew not to press her any more. As before, the matter was undoubtably closed.

After she had left us the following morning, Clara poured out her heart on paper.

My dear Jane,

I'm so sorry about last night. I must have seemed very odd. While thanking you for respecting my need to stop that conversation, I feel it right for me to explain a little by letter, to myself if not to you.

When I was alone in bed, your question kept echoing in my head. Why did praise make me confused of all things? Why can't I enjoy it as it's intended? I long to believe the praise in that letter I showed you, but not just his. Often people say nice things just casually, and I can't trust them. I look at their face to decide if they're really genuine, or I contradict any nice things they may say to me—I'm sure I only do so to test whether they've really meant what they've just said.

It's funny, you know. At first when I read your book, I was frustrated at those who had not known you well enough to see underneath your smiles and realize how you were, before you got to the point of collapsing. There was the frustration at others, because I know you and can read you (mostly!), but there was frustration at you, too, Jane. I thought, *Why didn't Jane say how ill she was?* Especially to the doctors, because you always got on with them so well. I even got irritated about that bit where you described how gaily you announced that you were "being unzipped again, folks!" but underneath you begged for someone to break through your role-playing, to sit down beside you and weep with you.

I have done that too, Jane. It wasn't until your penetrating questions last night that I consciously accepted that I, too, have hidden my own kind of pain. I understand now what you mean when you say everyone has pain. Some of us bury it so deep, we never dare to accept it. You touched on something very deep in me which I've never shared with anyone before. Well, I've never really allowed myself to think about it.

You see, I used to be praised about what a wonderful little girl I was. An uncle was particularly admiring. He used to come round to see Dad quite often. I hope you don't need me to explain exactly where all this led. When I was thirteen, he started to take me out for "treats." At first he took me hiking, but as I developed he started being interested in me. [Here there were crossings-out on the page.] I'm sorry, I can't explain more. It's too painful to recall it.

Every time he brought me back home, my mom or dad asked how I'd enjoyed myself. My uncle always used to rehearse it all beforehand: I was to tell of the views, the lochs, the walks. I longed for my parents to see the sham of those stories. I remember thinking, *Please, Mom, look at my eyes and don't listen to these words he told me to say.* But I didn't. I couldn't. I suppose they never questioned whether anything funny was going on.

I was reading an article in a magazine the other day which said that child abuse is *never* the child's fault. That really struck me. I suppose that's what has freed me enough to dare write all this to you now. I think I always blamed myself, even though at the time I had not known any way out. If he hadn't been my nice uncle, I could have said no. But as it was, I didn't know how to. I still blame myself for that, even though I felt forced into it. I don't know. I'm too mixed up about it.

You know, I hate people to blame the past for how they are now, but perhaps I shouldn't be so dismissive. I had never made this connection, but last night I found it only helpful to understand myself a little more. It helps to have discovered why, perhaps, I don't trust people naturally. Only those who look at my eyes. I feel I always have to put on a brave face—just as you felt you had to in your different pain.

This has all been so tightly locked up, nobody has ever known. Thank you for understanding as I know you will. That helps.

With my love,
Clara

Clara is not alone in hiding where she really hurts. It is hard to disclose our pain when others may not understand. To do so is to risk meeting a response which does not take time to understand and to care. It is to expose willingly the very hurt to be trampled on.

It is easier to say nothing, to talk only about pain which is acceptable to others and not necessarily about where we really hurt. Others may only ever glimpse that.

Mark was very different from Clara. When he came up to me at the end of a meeting, he did so with studied reluctance.

"I wish I'd never come," he lamented.

His friend looked embarrassed for my sake and wearied for himself. "But you said you wanted God's help," he reminded him.

Mark set his shoulders. "I need God to take me out of this dreadful situation." He was sure that his situation was so grim that the only way God could possibly help was by rescuing him from it.

He began to tell of his pain, giving more and more details and barely pausing for breath. He gave no time for reflection, although he did make strategic halts at those emotional parts of his story which lent themselves to expressions of pity. Such a barrage of words was very different from Clara's silence.

Or was it? The more Mark talked, the less worthwhile I felt our discussion to be. He could talk about hurt, yes, but as his tale went round and round, I sensed that he was touching only the periphery. I watched his face as he dangled his lurid details before me, waiting for my exclamations of sympathy. He seemed untouched even by the most pitiful things he was saying. Was he unable to face his pain? Using words to avoid thinking about what really hurt him?

Clara's suffering had helped her to understand others in a way which was so special that that was her hallmark as a nurse. Mark was not able to reach out to others yet. The discomfort he had expressed at the very outset was at hearing that others suffer as well. He did not like to accept that, because he had never really accepted his own pain. He felt that pain singled him out. He even rejected that his friend beside him wanted to help.

His friend caught my eye and shrugged hopelessly. He must have been faithful indeed to have stood by so demanding a person as Mark.

I searched for some reassurance to give him. "I'm sure your friends do care."

Mark countered me immediately. He spoke straight and directly. His words were a sweeping reproach.

"Everyone always tries to help," he said. "But they can't understand, so their 'answers' are never right."

I flinched. How many people like Mark had I unconsciously put off as I had tried to "help" them?

I began to feel very inadequate. The easiest way out seemed to be to blame him for being too selfish. It was the presence of his friend that kept me persevering. I did not want to disappoint him.

How would Jesus have shown Mark his love? I wondered rather desperately. I looked around the little room at the back of the church. Dusty pictures drooped over the peeling paint of the walls.

Certainly, any "answers" would have seemed intolerable to Mark without his seeing the compassion in Jesus' eyes. They would have seemed only to be a sign of others' inability to draw close to him in his pain.

Maybe Jesus would have met with Mark at church and would have been moved with compassion to touch him and heal him as he did the woman who was physically crippled (Luke 13). But on that occasion Jesus made some others in church feel "ashamed of themselves." Would he have been ashamed of my impoverished attempts to help now?

Maybe Jesus would have sat down with Mark and talked with him about yeast. He would have reminded him that he need only a tiny amount to cause a whole batch of heavy dough to be raised into light bread (Matthew 13). What was it my recipe book said at the top of the page on bread-making, I wondered slightly irreverently? I had read it often enough: "Yeast is that magic ingredient that changes a flat, lumpy cake of flour and water into something you'll hardly recognize." Would Jesus have promised Mark that he would be transformed in the same way when the Holy Spirit suffused him with new life? Undoubtedly that would have encouraged him, lifting him out of the heaviness of life in which he had become entrenched. But such inspiring "answers" usually came in parables.

Maybe Jesus would have grieved over Mark's stubborn self-pity, saying, "If you only knew today what is needed for peace! . . . You did not recognize the time when God came to save you!" (Luke 19:42,44, GNB) But he would not have spoken thus in judgment. As over Jerusalem, he would have been weeping . . . but not impotent tears because there was nothing He could do. Jesus' tears would have been shed because He knew He could help.

But Mark had closed himself off from any help other than to be lifted out of his furnace. He would not understand Jesus' tears. "If Jesus felt so upset about me, He would use His power to help me out of this mess," he reasoned. If he could not be helped as he wanted so adamantly, he would reject God. For years he had "confided" in people, seeking their help. But a bit of him hung back from any such help. He was curled around his own hurt and was afraid to risk being uncurled. A bit of him wanted to hug his hurt, to nurture and protect it. But his grief became his grievance.

I came home that night feeling drained and dejected. Mark had refused to let God into where he hurt, so there could never be any harvest. He saw his pain only as a waste.

I could not condemn him. The compassion of others is a relief at first and I had sought it myself. Occasionally, I too had "confided" in others, telling myself that I was merely obeying Jocelyn's advice. But I knew deep down that this was more than sharing with them. I wanted to convey to them my oppression as well. I wanted them to be oppressed with me, to show me that they understood. I interpreted events to conform to my own bitter outlook.

Whenever I allow myself such indulgent luxury, I lose any sense of God's peace. I feel alone. Others' pity slips through the soul as through a sieve, leaving a bitterness more stark than before. Then I want others to join me in feeling sorry for me. I say that I want them to pray for me. Actually I want them to feel for me too. I get it wrong. I demand too much. I allow my suffering to impose on others more than they are able to bear. I am tempted to pooh-pooh others' pain and say (to myself, if not out loud) that theirs is not as bad as mine.

"My situation is worse than that of Shadrach, Meshach and Abednego," I have said. "Others are singed, too."

But that is not true. It is a deceit. In speaking thus, I dishonor God. It is only those whom I drag in with me who are singed. It is I who have been put in this furnace. And, though I loathe the deceptively easy words, in fact God has protected me from being burned, as He has the children. And for Matthew, whose pain is to be so close to one who is suffering physically, his pathway is different from mine. The extent to which he is singed is part of his own relationship with his Lord.

Whenever I look at how grim I feel, I want to point to myself. That is not facing up to my pain. It is failing to accept it, and thereby failing to accept God in it. Sister Rachel, a nun whom Matthew and I have come to know and love dearly, once wrote of this as the pain of dying into life. "That is something we have to do alone with God," she wrote, and then, as if to earth her wisdom, she explained, "Others can and do help by being alongside us. Jesus took the disciples. He needed them, but they could not go all the way to the heart of His struggle and of course they fell asleep . . ."

It is only when I face my pain, and take the hand of my Lord in it, that I can reach out to others in a sincere and meaningful way. Only then do I see pain more from God's perspective. How "bad" the other person's pain is becomes irrelevant. Whenever we suffer, our Father suffers and grieves with us. He weeps over us. He never says, "Her pain is not as bad as mine."

The closer I come to my Lord, the more I am coming to see how my own pain—however extreme—only has any meaning in terms of His. For as I come nearer to Him, I see that what I am taught in my culture—that suffering is a sign of God's absence—is wrong. It is not so.

If I am to come close to God, I must encounter pain. For when Jesus showed His disciples bread at the Last Supper, He said, "This is my body." And He broke it. The Bread of Life was broken.

If I am to come close to God, then I will come close to His heart. And God's heart is not unfeeling, not free of pain. It is broken. God's heart bleeds. And more: It bleeds over me. It bleeds with pain because He loves me, more deeply than I ever imagine. His heart yearns for mine as a lover yearns for union with His bride. He yearns for my heart to beat in unison with His.

And what does He find instead? A heart of stone. Hard, cold and unyielding.

How God must be tempted to take my heart of stone and turn it into something which will satisfy His longings! For just as Jesus in the wilderness saw stones when He wanted bread, even now my Father sees stones: the stony hearts of His people whom He loves.

It is a temptation He resists. Instead He allows a gradual transformation. His yeast is at work: His Holy Spirit which suffuses me with His life, warming my coldness toward Him, lifting my heaviness.

And now I see that the stone is not something hard that a hard God holds out to me. The stone is in me. And God is a vulnerable God. He allows me to shout at Him for being hard, for giving me a hard stone when I want bread. He does not turn away. He stays open to accusation, misunderstanding and misinterpretation of His loving motives.

And so my Father's heart is full of pain. It is the pain of unfulfilled longing, the pain of loneliness. His is the pain of a broken relationship, of bereavement. His is the pain of a parent grieving over a child's handicap. For my lack of love is no less than a handicap when compared with the fullness of life and love which my Father constantly offers.

And I only ever glimpse God's own pain.

Stoneground Bread

He who supplies seed . . . and bread . . . will enlarge the harvest (2 Corinthians 9:10).

Three huge beech trees stand majestically on the far side of our garden wall. The sun is streaming through their widespread branches whose winter bareness scarcely filters its rays as they flood, dancing, into our living room. The unexpected shower of March snow earlier this morning has almost melted now, with only a smattering of white patches glistening and sparkling brightly on the lawn.

The double-glazing of the large patio windows serves to magnify the sun's warmth. It has brought a flush to my cheeks, relaxing them with a glow quite different from the pale, pinched sensation which accompanies severe pain. It is a welcome change from the past weeks of strain.

About half an hour ago, Matthew meandered

downstairs and wandered through from the kitchen. I remained where I was, strewn comfortably across two beanbags. My eyes were almost closed as I enjoyed a precious, child-free half-hour of quietness in which to be thoughtful.

Matthew, too, was very relaxed after his restful morning in bed on his day off. I flopped one arm around him as he bent over me and smiled.

"How are you?" he asked.

I did not want to talk about physical pain nor any symptoms I felt. In part, I wanted to be his wife, not his patient. Mostly, though, I knew that at that moment they seemed to be the least significant aspect of how I felt.

I chose to answer him differently. "I'm asking God to help me to accept how I am and to keep accepting it rather than feel sorry for myself." I paused, then realized that Matthew was waiting for me to say more.

"And I'm thanking Him for keeping my spirits up over the past weeks, and begging Him please to keep them up now." I met his steady gaze. "I'm frightened, Matthew. If I start thinking about the prognosis and getting depressed, I'll be sunk."

"Certainly," Matthew agreed quickly with the last comment. We were both quiet and thoughtful.

I have to readjust. My life, my activities, my thinking. It has been more than a year since that night when the surgeon decided to "watch and wait." They have watched my collapse at the health center, and calmly, it seemed, they waited to see if the time had come for yet another major operation. Thankfully, they got away with only a minor one.

Some things have changed. The intensity of the symptoms has diminished enough for the doctors to agree that I would be better to feel ill at home than in the hospital. The urgency for another major operation has faded now—postponed at least for a while, until perhaps I collapse once more.

But much is the same. Still they are watching and waiting until the day when they cannot avoid opening me up once again. Still, life seems a battle of will to keep going despite how my body feels. Still I am in pain and I feel sick, like the nausea of pregnancy but without the hope of release in a few months' time.

Could God want this? Could He have some purpose in it? It seems so mundane compared with the wonderful ways I see God working in others. Perhaps it's easy for me to see others' ministry because I only see the harvest, while their everyday business and battles against pain remain hidden to me.

I do not know the answers. But I am sure God knows that pain is bad. He cannot expect me to welcome pain, which is why He promises that it will soon end. In heaven will be the harvest from pain: the goodness which comes out of pain. There will be the fruit of God's Spirit in all its abundance. There will be the sensitivity, the understanding, the quiet self-giving I find in those who have suffered. In heaven we will see what we only glimpse now.

And I do know that God accepts everything I offer to Him. He takes my offering as a seed from which He brings forth His harvest. The warmth of today's sun reminds me that now it is springtime. Seedtime. So I am offering my present suffering to God, for Him to heal me or to be with me in it. I am offering myself to God to be used as He wants, offering my hands for God to do what He wants to do through them, however useless they seem to me.

Tentatively, I am reaching out to accept the stone which ongoing pain seems to be, and as I do so I see the hand of Him who gives. It is a hand so loving that it is scarred, hurting, bleeding for me. It is the hand of the One who is the Bread of Life.

Far from being a gloomy morning of resigned self-pity, this morning I feel freed to a new sense of joy. It is a solemn joy. It is the joy of accepting that there can be pain, tears, mourning over what might have been. It is the joy of hearing the question, "Do you believe in the goodness of God?" and knowing that no matter what, I do.

This prayer is not so much what I say to Him, but more about opening myself for Him to do what He wants in me. For I see that it is neither my successes nor my fruitfulness which are important in my life, but union with God. That is what He made me for.

This morning I see that to come close to His heart is to encounter pain. But with that pain there is the joy and privilege of my heart beating more closely to His own pulse. What anticipation there is for when such union becomes complete!

It was Matthew who broke our thoughtful silence. "Gosh, lady," he said. I looked round at his face questioningly. "That's profound," he concluded.

"No, it's not," I countered. "It's just ordinary. It's just everyday business—accepting oneself before God."

"Yes," came Matthew's pensive reply, "but your

everyday business is profound. It has to be, because of what's happening to you."

A flicker of pride could have welled up inside me as I let his words sink in. But I was too caught up in my reason for praying as I had been on this particular morning.

Matthew stood up and, his arms folded, he gazed outside. The sun had risen higher now, and against its silvery brightness some dark crows were silhouetted black and menacing.

"Those crows are terribly destructive," I remarked. "Look at them! They're pulling those poor trees to pieces."

As we watched, no fewer than four crows worked on different parts of the trees. They pecked with their beaks and stamped with their feet, clawing determinedly at the twigs until they had cut off the piece they wanted. Some of the twigs seemed enormous, and I wondered that they were not too heavy for the birds to be able to carry.

Matthew was more philosophical than I. "I was just thinking how clever it all is," he mused. "If you look carefully, they only take the bits which come off easily. It's a very neat way of removing the weak parts of the tree which actually has the effect of keeping the whole thing growing more strongly."

He was right.

And of course, the crows were not purposeless. Their tearing down is not futile. Elsewhere, they are building their nests. But the trees where the new nests are being built are half a mile away, out of my sight. From my beanbags, I can see only the destructive tearing down.

How easy it is to mourn when I see tearing down, to fail to see that that is part of building. It cannot, or should not, be separated from building up. For without the tearing down of twigs, there would be no building of nests.

Which is why I'm uncomfortable to talk about the destructive element of my suffering. I may feel only the brokenness in my own suffering. I may never see what is being built up. The harvest is only glimpsed now. Indeed, I have no certainty that I will ever see the harvest from my pain. But that does not—or should not—matter. Indeed, just as the crows' new nests are not even in the same tree as these ones where twigs are being torn off, perhaps the harvest from my pain may not be visible in my life here, but it may yet be to come. Or perhaps others may see what I cannot.

But of one thing I am certain. In God's timing it will be there, like the new nests in the trees half a mile away.

"As long as the earth endures, seedtime and harvest . . . will never cease" (Genesis 8:22).

Real Help
for Real Hurts

Quantity   Total

___   **A PATHWAY THROUGH PAIN** by Jane Grayshon. How $___
       to press on with joy despite chronic pain and suffering. A
       sensitive and insightful book. ISBN 0-89840-291-3/$8.99

___   **WHEN YOUR DREAMS DIE** by Marilyn Willett Heavilin. $___
       Practical advice for finding strength and hope through
       life's major disappointments. ISBN 0-89840-268-9/$7.99

___   **FINDING THE HEART TO GO ON** by Lynn Anderson. $___
       A beautifully written learning experience from the life
       of David. Discover the source of his strength.
       ISBN 0-89840-309-X/$8.99

___   **DON'T JUST STAND THERE, PRAY SOMETHING** by $___
       Ronald Dunn. An inspiring look at how you can pray with
       greater purpose and power—for your own needs as well
       as the needs of others. ISBN 0-89840-312-X/$7.99

**Your Christian bookseller should have these products in stock.
Please check with him before using this "Shop by Mail" Form.**

Send completed order form to: **HERE'S LIFE PUBLISHERS, INC.**
                              P. O. Box 1576
                              San Bernardino, CA 92402-1576

Name _____

Address _____

City _____ State _____ Zip _____

| Payment enclosed | **ORDER TOTAL** $___
    (check or money order only) | **SHIPPING and
| Visa | Mastercard | HANDLING** $___
#_____ | ($1.50 for one item,
Expiration Date _____ | $0.50 for each additional.
Signature _____ | Do not exceed $4.00.)
                                       | **APPLICABLE
       For faster service, | SALES TAX (CA 6.75%) $___
        call toll free:
        1-800-950-4457** | **TOTAL DUE** $___

Please allow 2 to 4 weeks for delivery.
Prices subject to change without notice.